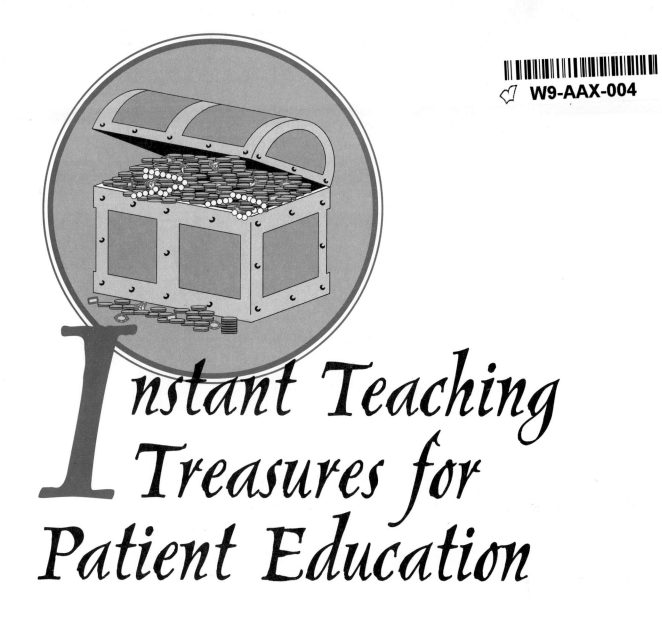

Instant Teaching Treasures for Patient Education

Instant Teaching Treasures for Patient Education

Gaye Ragland

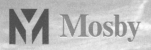

Mosby

St. Louis   Baltimore   Boston   Carlsbad   Chicago   Naples   New York   Philadelphia   Portland
London   Madrid   Mexico City   Singapore   Sydney   Tokyo   Toronto   Wiesbaden

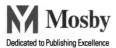
Dedicated to Publishing Excellence

A Times Mirror
Company

Vice President and Publisher: Jacqueline Katz
Editor: Laurie Stahl
Developmental Editor: Barbara Watts
Editing, Production, and Design: Graphic World Publishing Services
Manufacturing Manager: Betty Richmond

1st EDITION
Copyright © 1997 by Mosby-Year Book, Inc.

Printed in the United States of America
Composition by Graphic World, Inc.
Lithography/color film by Graphic World, Inc.
Printing/binding by Courier

Mosby-Year Book, Inc.
11830 Westline Industrial Drive
St. Louis, Missouri 63146

Library of Congress Cataloging in Publication Data

Ragland, Gaye.
     Instant teaching treasures for patient education / Gaye Ragland.
        p.   cm.
     Includes bibliographical references.
     ISBN 0-8151-4699-X
        1. Patient education—Handbooks, manuals, etc.   I. Title.
        [DNLM: 1. Patient Education—methods—nurses' instruction.
2. Teaching Materials.   W 85 R143 i   1996]
RT90.R34   1997
614.5′07—dc20
DNLM/DLC
for Library of Congress   96-29271
                                                                      CIP

ISBN 0-8151-4699-X
96 97 98 99 00 / 9 8 7 6 5 4 3 2 1

Contributors

Mary Ann Canterbury, RN, MSN
Instructor
University of Mississippi School of Nursing
Jackson, MS

DeBrynda B. Davey, RN, EdD
Associate Professor
Director, Undergraduate Program
University of Mississippi School of Nursing
Jackson, MS

Paul A. Davey, M.S., LPC
Child Psychotherapist
Adolescent, Child and Family Clinic
Jackson, MS

Bonnie Davis, RN, DNS
Associate Professor
University of Mississippi School of Nursing
Jackson, MS

LaVerne Grant, RN, MS
Instructor
University of Mississippi School of Nursing
Jackson, MS

Nancy Hollis, RN, MSN
Instructor
University of Mississippi School of Nursing
Jackson, MS

Susan Lofton, RN, MSN
Instructor
University of Mississippi School of Nursing
Jackson, MS

Billie Phillips, RN, MSN
Instructor
University of Mississippi School of Nursing
Jackson, MS

Reviewers

May L. Duncan, RN, BSN, MPA
Instructor
Haney Technical Center
Panama City, FL

Martha Jones, RN
General Manager
AccuCare Home Health of Arlington
Columbia Homecare Group
Arlington, TX

Stacy Reel, RN, BSN
Education Coordinator
Haney Technical Center
Panama City, FL

About the Author

Gaye Ragland, RN, BSN has been a practicing Registered Nurse for over twenty years. As a dean's list scholar, she graduated from University of Mississippi School of Nursing in 1975. Her love for patient teaching began there with her first job as a student nurse working in the newborn nursery caring for well babies and helping teach new mothers.

Following graduation Gaye worked in long term care for nearly a decade. She practiced in roles ranging from Staff Nurse to Director of Nursing Services. During those years she taught patients, staff, and families. The next career turn took her to a certified nursing assistant program where she was an instructor and eventually Director of Education for more than four years. This was the time in her career that her love for teaching flourished.

From classroom teaching Gaye moved into a staff development position in a fast-growing home health agency. Very soon thereafter she was called on to develop practical, "user-friendly" patient teaching tools for homecare nurses with whom she worked. In 1991 Gaye was voted by her own colleagues as Professional Support Staff of the Year. She was named Mississippi Nursing Association's District 13 Nurse Educator II of the Year in 1992 and 1994. She was honored by Mosby Resource Applications in 1993 as the recipient of the national Thelma A. Schorr Award for innovations and creativity in staff development. In 1994 Gaye was presented the Fredrick Rogers/J. Dudley Westbrook Award by the Mississippi Association of Homecare for promotion of the homecare industry in Mississippi. The same year Gaye received the Distinguished Service Award for Health Promotion from the Mississippi Joint Conference on Aging.

In May 1996, Gaye completed serving a four year gubernatorial appointment to the Mississippi State Board of Nursing Home Administrators. She is on the advisory board for Mosby's *Home Health Focus* newsletter. In addition, she is on the Board of Review for the journal, *Home Care Provider.* Gaye serves as Education Consultant with Sta-Home Health Agency, Jackson, Mississippi.

Gaye's conference sessions all end with the same slide:

"You Can't Burn Out If You Ain't Lit Up In The First Place."

And after attending one of her sessions, participants leave more lit up than they ever thought possible. She jokes, juggles, and plays kazoos. But most of all she shares a love for her profession and a commitment to patient teaching. She reminds nurses that knowledge gained must be knowledge shared, thus awakening the "teacher" within.

Today Gaye has become a popular national nursing speaker with speaking engagements too numerous to list. She travels throughout the country lighting fires in nurses who are struggling to find the time and tools needed for patient teaching. For many nurses, job demands are so great that finding time for patient teaching is only a dream. For others, limited resources decelerate the process. But with the chest of treasures to follow, knowledge can be shared in a way that is quick, creative, meaningful, and fun. And patient teaching dreams *will* become realities.

Preface

Teaching becomes one of the primary vehicles for the promotion of wellness once the patient is able to take in new information. There are so many ingredients that must be addressed in the plan of care including medications, diet, mobility orders, equipment, infection control, and the list goes on and on. Without a thorough understanding of each of these aspects of care, the patient's ability to actively participate in a quest for improvement is quite compromised.

Though most healthcare professionals desire to share in the patient's drive for improvement, inadequate staffing often results in little or no time for patient teaching. But for other professionals who have the time, practical resources may be the cause of the patient teaching deficit.

If patient teaching material is to be useful, it must meet the needs of both the patient and the professional. It must be "user friendly." It must be organized in a way that the patient understands. Teaching material must be non-threatening, therefore motivating the patient to seek more information instead of turning away from that which is offered. And it is with the gaining of more information that the patient will be better positioned to make quality life choices leading to improved patient outcomes.

Though nobody has a perfectly accurate prediction of the future of healthcare, many believe that financial restraints on our system for years to come will limit allowable patient visits. Most envision providers continuing to care for the same types of patients with the same types of diagnoses. But for the real "clincher": healthcare professionals will be expected to do so with records of improved patient outcomes. How will we accomplish **more with less?**

 Pages with this symbol can be copied. These "instant patient teaching treasures" will enable the teacher to make patient teaching fun. These treasured gems will empower the teacher to stimulate the patient to think critically and ease the documentation burdens faced by all. Optional suggestions give the teacher ideas to liven selected sessions with icons and laughter. Each exercise is ready for quick and easy use. Cash them in today for improved patient results. The treasures are buried no more!

> This text is intended as a resource and educational aid. The content is intended to supplement, not substitute for, the advice of the patient's physician. The patient's physician should be consulted before the patient embarks on any new program or makes any changes in a current program.

Acknowledgments

Thank you, Mosby, for inviting me to take this wild and wonderful journey. Thank you Jackie Katz and Laurie Stahl for associating me with the idea for this book. It was truly my "lucky" day when I first met you both at Staff Development '94 in Las Vegas. And how could I ever say an adequate thanks to my developmental editor, Barb Watts, whose soothing voice talked me through many anxiety attacks. I really do want to make good on my offer of catfish and turnip greens.

Thank you to the faculty members at University of Mississippi School of Nursing who contributed additional treasures for the book. You quickly responded and so ably shared from your wealth of knowledge and experience. My trips to meet with you at the school revived many memories of my student days at UMC. And with those memories alive and well, a special thank you to Helen Jones, Kaye Milhorn, and Bobbie Ward. As faculty members teaching this young married student who took time out to have her baby, each of you played an important part in my life as you encouraged me to resume my studies. At the time it didn't seem so significant. Twenty years later, I realize the level of your commitment to the future of your students.

A special thank you to Belinda Patterson. You always had time to hear my ideas. Then you made sure I had everything I needed to see them through. And Rebecca Askew, thank you for promoting me and inspiring me to write. You will always be a mentor to me.

Thank you to my many friends who offered encouragement along the way. A very special thanks to Wayne Clark for your sacrifice at holiday time to see that my office was quickly operational. Thanks to my friends at Wynndale who asked me every Sunday, "How's it coming along?" Thank you Christie, Nancy, and Cindy. Everybody needs good friends. And how could I ever say an adequate thank you to you, Glynda. This is my chance to tell the world that "I am *your* raving fan!" It is my dream that we will work together again.

Susan, I'm so fortunate to have a "nurse sister" like you. What a special bond we share. Thanks to you and Julianne for your good ideas. Thank you, Mother, who along with Daddy, insisted that we get a good education. I wish you, Mom, could have been a nurse. You would have been the best. And a special thanks to Mom's home health nurse, Sally Shaw. Your attention to Mom enabled me to spend more time writing. You exemplify excellence in your practice every day. And last but not least, my deepest thanks to my best friend and husband, Tim, and our daughters, Rana (the world's greatest first grade teacher) and Katie Jane (the future ER physician). It was so important to each of you that I had everything I needed and was never disturbed. You cooked and cleaned and ate many, many pizzas. You, my family, are *my* treasures. I dedicate this book to you.

A Look Inside the Treasure Chest

Resources

Teaching Treasures to Keep on Hand

- A selection of hats that identify the various roles of the caregiver
- Straight pins
- Rubber ducky (squeaky toy)
- Pens, pencils
- Black pen
- Red markers
- 4 black markers
- Orange marker
- Blunt-end scissors
- Bar of soap and washcloth
- Red stars
- Red sticky dots
- Stop watch
- Insulin syringe
- Old shoe
- Tape
- Magazines (food pictures)
- 4-6 labels from perishable food items (Meat labels for poultry, beef, pork, and product expiration dates)
- 3 labels from sugar-containing foods
- Red food coloring
- Teaspoon
- Orange stick/nail file
- Paper towels
- Clean towel
- Medication set-up device
- Empty egg carton
- Current medication reference book
- Small rewards
- Ribbon 3" in length (2 bright colors)
- Wire rimmed glasses
- Large brimmed hat
- Hot glue gun (optional)

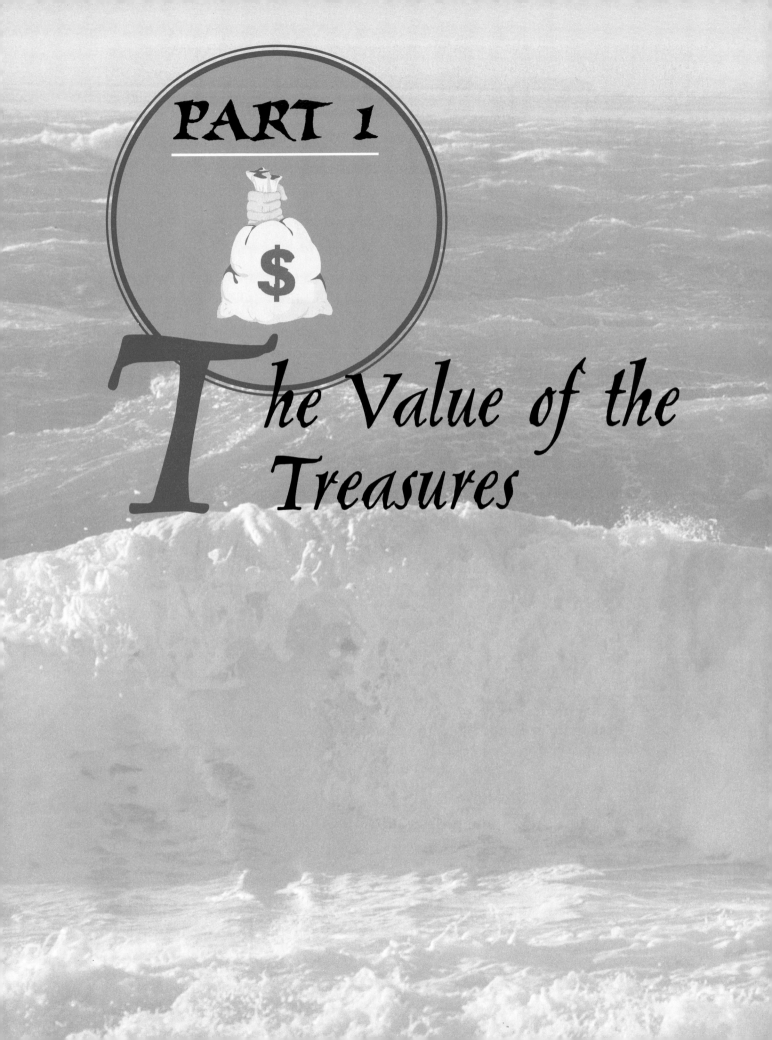

PART 1

The Value of the Treasures

THE VALUE OF THE TREASURES

Compact and Copy Ready

As a changing healthcare system bursts forth before our eyes, never have the challenges been greater to accomplish better outcomes in fewer visits while keeping costs low and quality high. Whether healthcare is delivered at the hospital bedside, rural clinic treatment room, or kitchen table of the homecare patient, easy to transport and ready to use creative teaching materials are both a necessity and a luxury. *Instant Teaching Treasures for Patient Education* is portable and ready to copy. And of course, photocopying is permitted if copied for use by the "teacher" who owns this book.

User "Friendly"

Instant Teaching Treasures for Patient Education is easy to use and geared to meet the individualized needs of special patients. Included are instructions for the use of each teaching treasure, suggestions for selected visual aids to enhance the learning process, exercise options that can add fun, "educator insights" that offer helpful hints and special reminders for the teacher, and answer keys to check your patient's work. There are pictures and cartoons that are ideal for the patient who has limited reading and writing skills. This collection of teaching treasures has something for everyone.

Necessary For The Patient

Have you ever had surgery? If so, do you remember that physician visit when the doctor was explaining the procedure you were about to undergo? You had questions. The doctor had answers. The pamphlets you probably received were loaded with information and instructions that provided much needed assurance.

Because of the trust relationship between the patient and professional caregiver, the strategy for providing patient reassurance begins with the sharing of information through quality patient teaching. Some patients take in new information with a positive anticipation. Others may face the future with dread. But regardless of the reaction, a better understanding of the patient's own condition affords the patient the opportunity for good decision making leading to improved patient outcomes. It is essential that we share what we know.

Helps The Caregiver At Home

There are many patients whose future rests in the helping hands of their dedicated caregivers. Caregivers often struggle as they attempt to practice this "art of caregiving" without formal training. Many never receive a caregiver class on body mechanics. Most caregivers did not have the opportunity to attend those early nursing school classes on tissue hypoxia and what happens when patients are not properly positioned. Unfortunately, their learning often takes place after the back injury or well into the breakdown of their loved one's fragile skin.

If we expect improved patient outcomes in fewer actual visits, "mini" nursing school classes must take place at the bedside, in treatment rooms and around kitchen tables. *Instant Teaching Treasures for Patient Education* includes many jewels for the caregiver including a variety of motivational gems. It also contains nuggets for teaching signs of exhaustion and overload. When will your next "mini" nursing class take place?

Validates Teaching

With a host of industry regulations, patient teaching is yet another area that is subject to scrutiny. *Instant Teaching Treasures for Patient Education* is designed to be copied and used in locations where the patients are. For the hospital or clinic patient, the treasures will be given to the patient to take home. For the homecare patient they will be used during the visit and then left in the home. What better evidence of quality patient teaching?

Stimulates Critical Thinking

The successful dieter says, "I was successful this time because I made my mind up to do it!" The now non-smoker says, "I quit this time for me!" Medical professionals continually watch patients make decisions: major, minor, good, and bad. Reflecting back to the days of choosing a college, the good choice came only after gathering data about all the possibilities. Likewise, patients need understandable data as they endeavor to make good choices that yield positive and often life-changing outcomes. Since many patients have limited physical and financial resources from which to draw information, they depend on the medical professional to deliver information as a part of the delivery of healthcare. And with *Instant Teaching Treasures for Patient Education,* the professional must only reach inside this chest for the treasure that will enable the patient to make the most precious of choices.

Eases the Documentation Burden

After the teacher shares the photocopied teaching treasures with the patient, the original treasures will remain intact and a part of this reference book. As the content taught is documented in the patient's medical record, this easy to use text will be both a reminder of what was taught and a planning tool for future patient teaching sessions.

Adds Joy To Your Daily Practice

It has been said that a wise teacher makes learning a joy and a joyful teacher is one who sees the fruits of the labor. The fruit may be the nod of a patient's head in response to new information. It may be the look of amazement when understanding of new information has just taken place. Ultimately, it is watching the patient gain or regain control because of active participation in the plan of care.

Laugh, listen, and learn together. Celebrate the victories. Try again when there are failures. Reschedule teaching time if the patient is too sick to concentrate. Bend with flexibility. Teach that which is most urgent first. Don't try to teach too much at once. Meet the patient where the patient is academically. And most of all, teach and reassure the patient in those areas in which there is a knowledge deficit causing the patient to feel scared and insecure.

With *Instant Teaching Treasures for Patient Education* the jewels are in hand for adding fun, challenges, and creativity to the lessons. So now open the treasure chest and appraise their worth!

PART 2

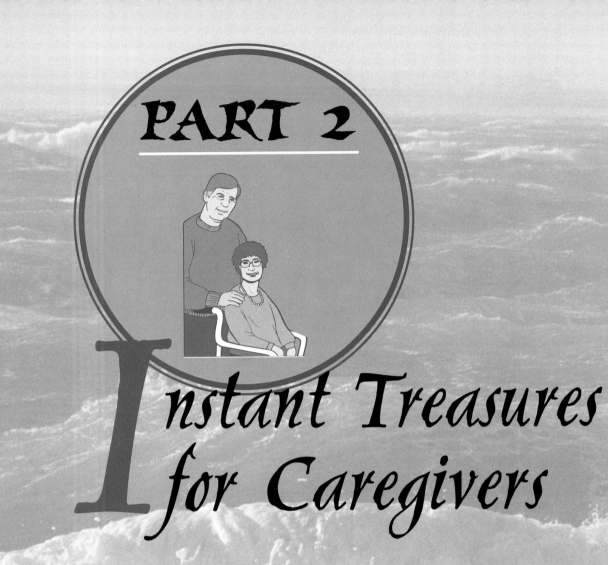

Instant Treasures for Caregivers

"HATS OFF" TO THE CAREGIVER

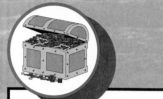

Treasure Chest

"Caregiver Storm Warning"

"Self-Care Tips to the Caregiver"

"Hats Off" sheet

Hat (of any kind)

Certificate

Pen or pencil with an eraser

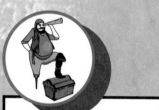

Educator Insights

Encourage the caregiver to verbalize frustrations and anxieties about the caregiving role. Talk about the positive aspects of caregiving as well. Look for areas to offer the caregiver both support and praise.

PREPARATION

1. Copy "Caregiver Storm Warning."
2. Copy "Hats Off to the Caregiver."
3. Review and copy "Self-Care Tips to the Caregiver."
4. Copy a "Caregiver" certificate.
5. Obtain a hat to use as an icon while discussing the various "hats" worn by the caregiver (i.e., cook, nurse, driver, etc.).
6. Make sure the caregiver has a pen or pencil.

IMPLEMENTATION

1. Explain to the caregiver the directions for completing the "Caregiver Storm Warning."
2. Have the caregiver complete the "Caregiver Storm Warning."
3. Point out and discuss danger areas.
4. Present and discuss "Self Care Tips to the Caregiver."
5. Encourage discussion of the "Hats Off" page. Set the hat icon on the table in front of the caregiver or have the caregiver hold the hat as you discuss the various roles. List additional hats worn by the caregiver in the box at the bottom of the page.
6. Present the caregiver with the selected certificate.
7. Leave "Self Care Tips" and "Hats Off" with the patient's caregiver.
8. Do not leave "Caregiver Storm Warning" in the patient's home.

By: Gaye Ragland RN BSN

CAREGIVER STORM WARNING

Directions: Answer the following questions by marking the best answer in the columns to the right.

	Always	Sometimes	Never	Rarely
1. I am the only person in the world in this situation.				
2. Nothing I do is ever enough.				
3. I feel all alone.				
4. I always seem to be exhausted.				
5. I resent my present situation.				
6. Caregiving responsibilities are now interfering with my work/social life.				
7. I never have a chance to be alone.				
8. I never get time just for me.				
9. I'm overeating.				
10. I never think of myself; that would be selfish.				
11. I no longer feel good about myself.				
12. There are no more happy times.				

7

"HATS OFF" TO THE CAREGIVER

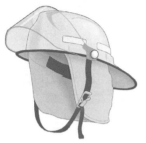

FIREMAN'S HAT
(Provides A Safe Environment)

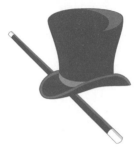

MAGICIAN'S HAT
(Keeps Everyone Happy)

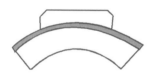

NURSE'S HAT
(Gives Patient Care)

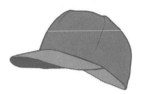

BASEBALL PLAYER'S HAT
(Provides Entertainment)

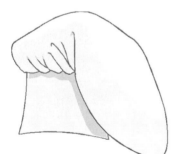

CHEF'S HAT
(Prepares Meals)

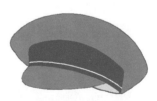

TAXI DRIVER'S HAT
(Provides Transportation)

OTHER HATS: _____ _____

_____ _____

_____ _____

"HATS OFF" TO THE CAREGIVER ANSWER SHEET:

OTHER HATS: Maid's Hat <u>   </u> (cleans the house)<u>   </u>

Dress Hat <u>   </u> (shops for food, medicine, etc.)<u>   </u>

Accountant's Hat <u>   </u> (balances finances and handles insurance)<u>   </u>

Maintenance Man's Hat (keeps the home in good working order)<u>   </u>

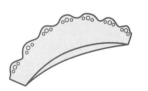

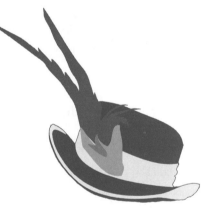

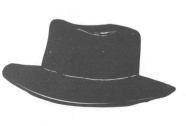

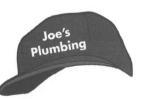

9

SELF-CARE TIPS FOR THE CAREGIVER

Practice the following tips as you strive to maintain balance in your life:

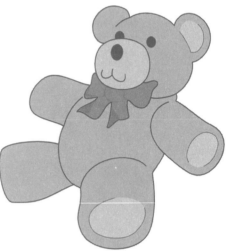

1. Don't have the "martyr" complex.

2. Accept help when family members or friends offer.

3. Don't mind asking for help when you need it.

4. Remember that asking for help in no way means you failed. It does mean you recognize and accept your limitations, and you want the best for your loved one.

5. Make sure you get enough rest. Caregiving is tiring at best.

6. Set realistic expectations. The solutions to many of the problems you face may be out of your control. If you could solve them you would.

7. Learn all you can about the disease that affects your loved one.

8. Know that guilt feelings are common.

9. Stay physically fit. Regular physical exams are a must.

10. Don't try to solve too many problems all at once. Deal with problems "little by little."

11. Don't let old promises or guilt "eat" at you.

10

12. Realize that some people will help more than others.

13. Be nice to yourself. A trip out to dinner or to the hairdresser can give you a new lease on life.

14. Plan for "time off." It may never happen unless you plan it.

15. Maintain friendships/relationships.

16. Eat a well balanced diet.

17. Keep laughter in your life.

18. Talk to someone who will listen . . . a friend, pastor, neighbor, or nurse.

19. Plan for the future when you will no longer be caring for your loved one. This will help make the adjustment easier when the time comes.

20. Set short-term goals. Celebrate Victories!

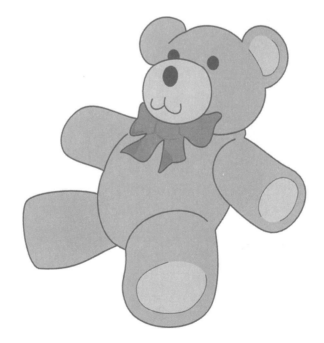

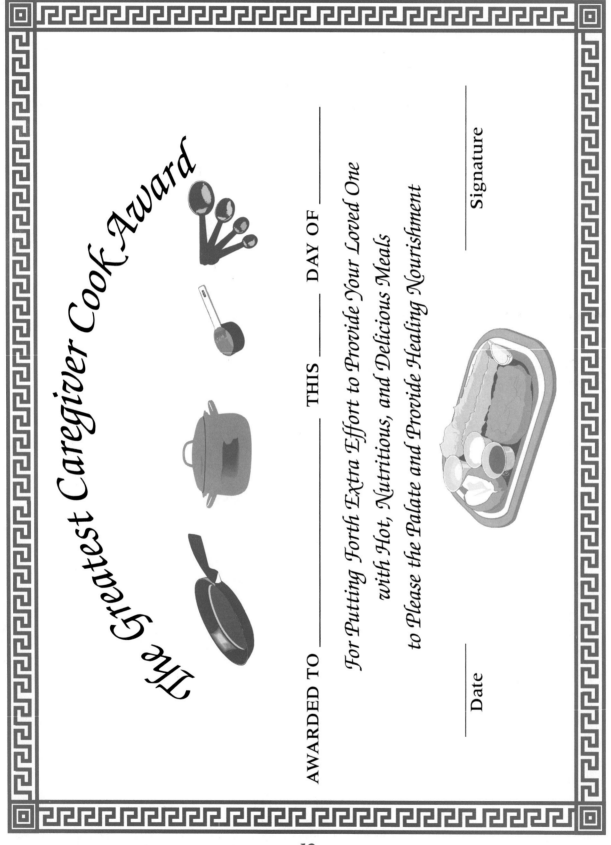

The Greatest Caregiver Cook Award

AWARDED TO _____

THIS _____ **DAY OF** _____

For Putting Forth Extra Effort to Provide Your Loved One
with Hot, Nutritious, and Delicious Meals
to Please the Palate and Provide Healing Nourishment

_____
Signature

_____
Date

12

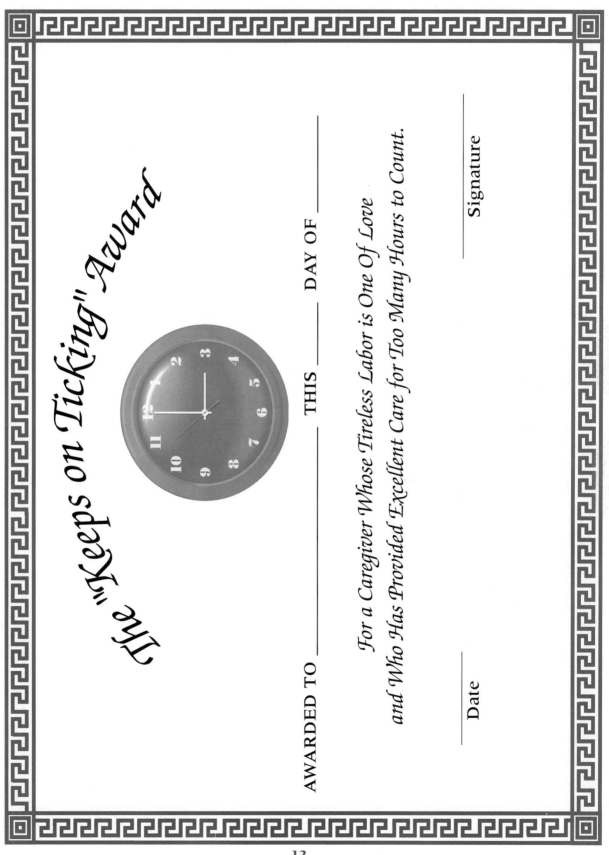

The "Keeps on Ticking" Award

AWARDED TO —————————————————

THIS ——— **DAY OF** ———

For a Caregiver Whose Tireless Labor is One Of Love and Who Has Provided Excellent Care for Too Many Hours to Count.

——————
Date

——————
Signature

13

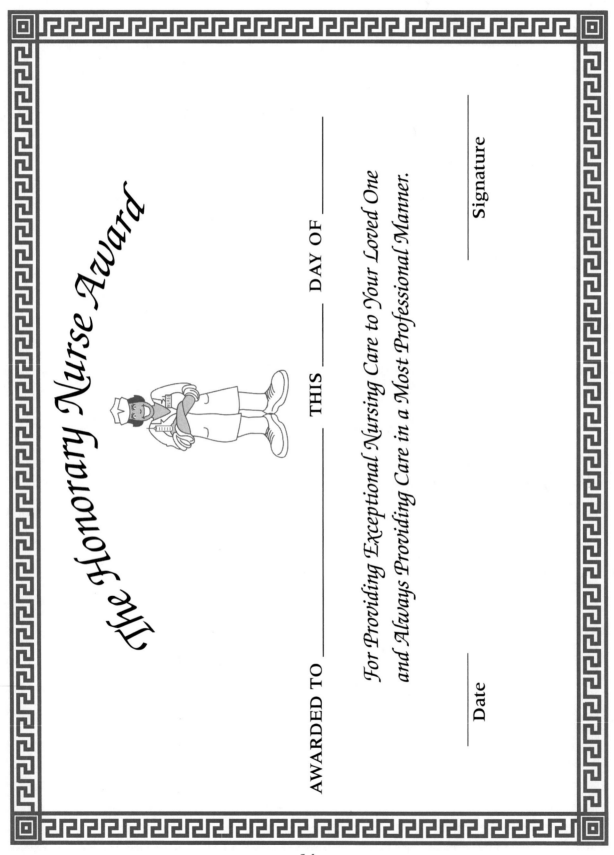

The Honorary Nurse Award

AWARDED TO _____ THIS _____ DAY OF _____

For Providing Exceptional Nursing Care to Your Loved One and Always Providing Care in a Most Professional Manner.

_____
Date

_____
Signature

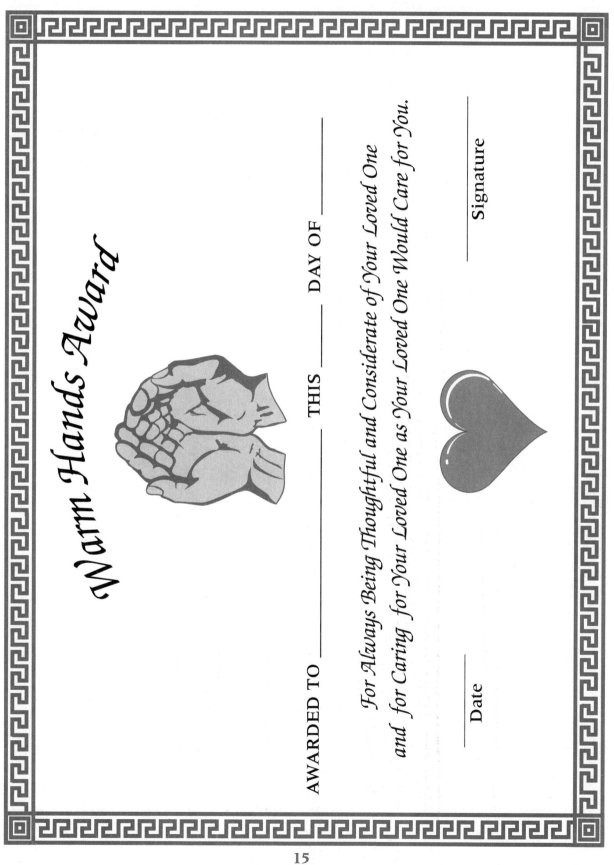

Warm Hands Award

AWARDED TO _____

THIS _____ **DAY OF** _____

For Always Being Thoughtful and Considerate of Your Loved One
and for Caring for Your Loved One as Your Loved One Would Care for You.

_____
Signature

_____
Date

15

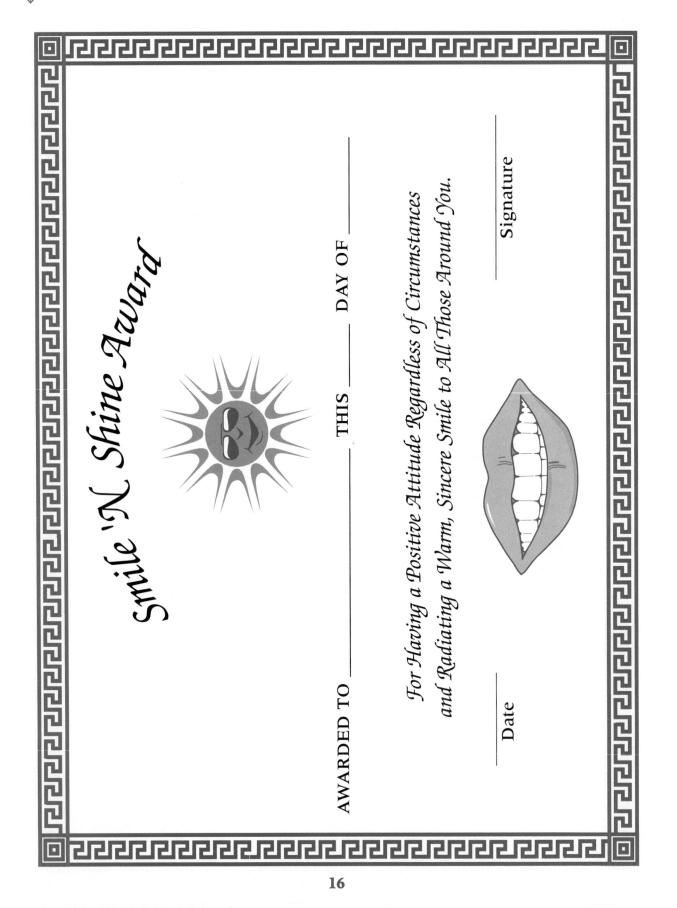

Smile 'N Shine Award

AWARDED TO

THIS _____ DAY OF _____

For Having a Positive Attitude Regardless of Circumstances and Radiating a Warm, Sincere Smile to All Those Around You.

_____
Date

_____
Signature

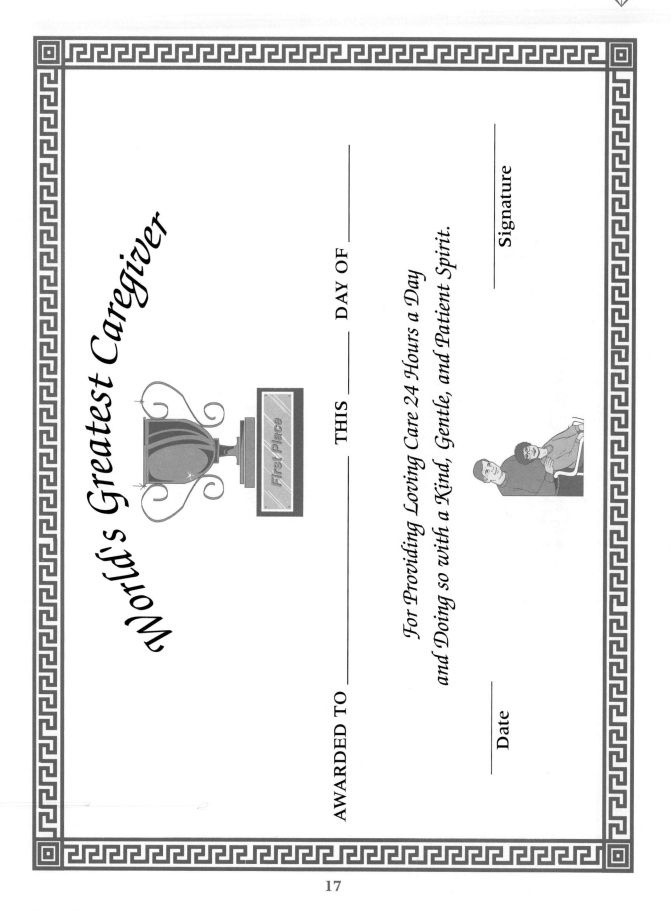

World's Greatest Caregiver

First Place

AWARDED TO _____

THIS _____ DAY OF _____

For Providing Loving Care 24 Hours a Day
and Doing so with a Kind, Gentle, and Patient Spirit.

Date _____

Signature _____

17

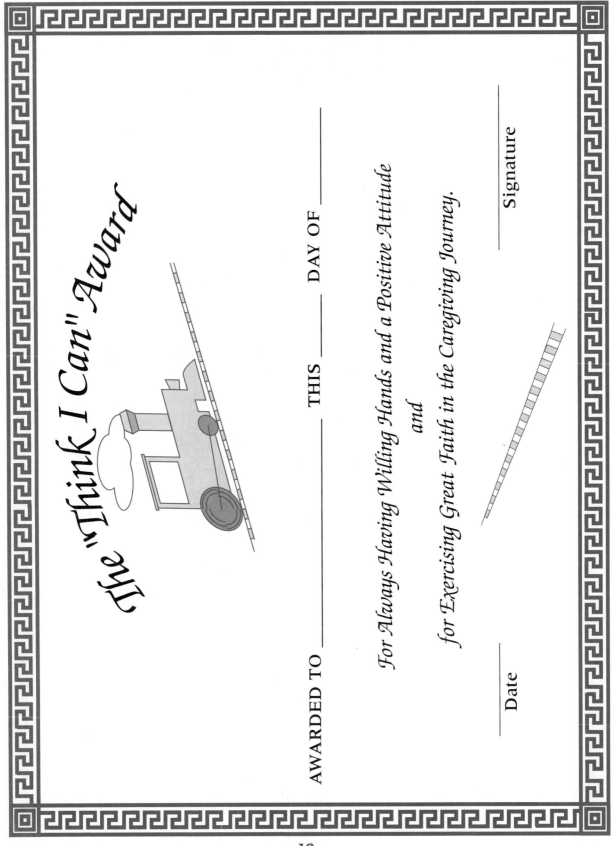

The "Think I Can" Award

AWARDED TO _____

THIS _____ DAY OF _____

For Always Having Willing Hands and a Positive Attitude

and

for Exercising Great Faith in the Caregiving Journey.

_____
Date

_____
Signature

18

"YOUR JUST REWARDS"

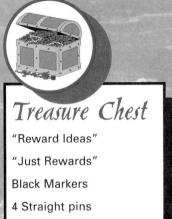

REWARDING
SPECIAL
PEOPLE

Treasure Chest

"Reward Ideas"

"Just Rewards"

Black Markers

4 Straight pins

1 Pair blunt-end scissors

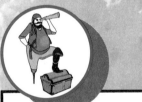

Educator Insights

Discuss with the patient the benefit that will come to him/her and to the specially recognized person.

PREPARATION

1. Review and copy "Reward Ideas."
2. Review and copy "Just Rewards." Suggestion: Copy "Just Rewards" on heavy weight paper.

IMPLEMENTATION

1. Assist the patient to identify person(s) who have helped in special ways. Discuss various ways of letting those persons know how special they are to the patient. "Reward Ideas" may be used as an example sheet when assisting the patient to determine award content.
2. Using "Reward Ideas," assist the patient in writing an acknowledgment to the special person(s).
3. With the black marker, write the person's name on the badge. Assist the patient to write a special message to that person (like "I Love You!").
4. Assist the patient to cut out the badge and pin it on the special person.

By: Paul A. Davey, M.S., LPC
Debrynda B. Davey, Ed.D., RN

REWARD IDEAS

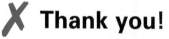

I Love You!

✗ Thank you for . . .

✗ I appreciate . . .

✗ You are special because . . .

✗ You deserve . . .

✗ I delight in your . . .

✗ Opportunity knocks! . . .

✗ Awaken your spirit with . . .

✗ . . . to your heart's content

✗ You'll enjoy . . .

✗ You'll love . . .

✗ . . . will revive your senses!

✗ You're the Best!

✗ You Deserve the Best!

✗ No One Beats You!

✗ I love you!

✗ You're a Winner!

✗ You are Remarkable!

✗ Especially for You!

✗ You are Perfect!

✗ Thank you!

✗ You Can Do It!

JUST REWARDS

TREASURE YOURSELF

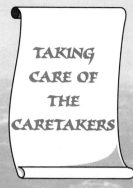

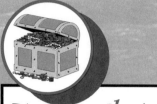

Treasure Chest

"Treasure Yourself"

"Respite Treasure Hunt"

Pen or pencil with an eraser

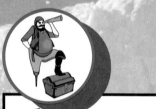

Educator Insights

If caretakers do not make time for respite, eventually their own physical and mental health will begin to suffer and it will impact the manner in which they care for their loved one. Remind your caretakers to treasure themselves and help them find a way to get the time they need and deserve.

PREPARATION

1. Review and copy "Treasure Yourself."
2. Review and copy "Respite Treasure Hunt."
3. Make sure the caretaker has a pen or pencil with an eraser.

IMPLEMENTATION

1. Discuss the importance of rest and relaxation activities, as well as the physical and psychological benefits.
2. Review possible respite activities with the caretaker. Use the teaching treasure "Treasure Yourself!" to start the discussion.
3. Assist the caretaker to determine at least one respite activity goal that is realistic and feasible. Use the teaching treasure "Respite Treasure Hunt" to plan goals and steps for achieving each step of the plan.
4. Reevaluate and revise the plan on a regular and as needed basis.
5. Leave "Treasure Yourself" with the patient's caregiver.

By: Debrynda B. Davey, Ed.D., RN
Paul A. Davey, MS, LPC

Treasure Yourself!

Ways to Recapture Pleasure

✗ Do something activating each week to remind yourself that not everyone is homebound (exercise or sports).

✗ Schedule a day out of the house each week.

✗ Open blinds and curtains on sunny days. Take in a few rays!

✗ Read something that is not work-related.

✗ Rent an action-adventure movie.

✗ Soak in a warm bath.

✗ Get a massage.

✗ Pay attention to your physical needs.

✗ Work in your garden or yard.

✗ Arrange for a sitter and sleep late once a week.

Respite Treasure Hunt

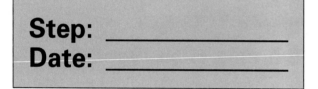

Goal: _____
Date: _____

Step: _____
Date: _____

Step: _____
Date: _____

Step: _____
Date: _____

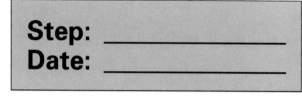

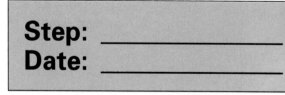

GOAL

3

2

1

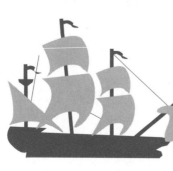

24

READY . . . AIM . . . APPETITE

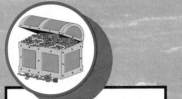

Treasure Chest

"How To Spice Up The Appetite"

"Ready . . . Aim . . . Appetite"

Pen or pencil with an eraser

Educator Insights

Keep the patient's special dietary needs and restrictions in mind as you work with the caregiver.

PREPARATION

1. Copy and review, "How To Spice Up Your Appetite."
2. Copy "Ready . . . Aim . . . Appetite."
3. Make sure the caregiver has a pen or pencil with an eraser.

IMPLEMENTATION

1. Read "How To Spice Up Your Appetite" with the caregiver.
2. Identify ideas from "Spice" sheet that the caregiver may use to try and improve the patient's appetite.
3. You *and* the caregiver list specific ideas on "Ready . . . Aim . . . Appetite" sheet, one in each ring, above the words "GOOD APPETITE."
4. Ask the caregiver to keep the target sheet in a conspicuous place (i.e., on the refrigerator).
5. Explain to the caregiver that you and the caregiver will total points for efforts made at the next visit.
6. Leave "How to Spice Up the Appetite" with the caregiver.

By: Gaye Ragland, RN, BSN

HOW TO SPICE UP THE APPETITE

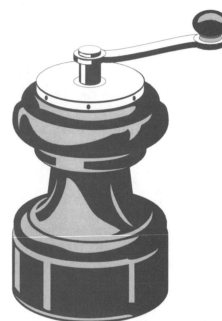

1. Encourage the patient to rest before mealtime.

2. Give mouth and tongue care a few minutes before the meal is served.

3. Eliminate unpleasant odors from the room in which the patient will eat. Cover suction bottles or any other equipment that may be unpleasant to the eyes.

4. Speak positively about the meal you are about to serve the patient.

5. Add seasonings according to the patient's preference but within limitations of the prescribed diet.

6. Sprinkle several drops of your loved one's favorite flavoring (orange or lemon, for example) on a cotton ball. Place the cotton ball in the room with the patient a few minutes before the meal is served. The pleasant aroma will often arouse the patient's interest in food and stimulate his desire to eat.

7. Have a designated place for the patient to sit at mealtime.

8. Make the table setting pleasant. Use colorful placemats, flowers, and bright dishes.

9. Serve the patient foods in a rich variety of tastes, colors, and textures. Arrange the food attractively on the plate. Make the setting a pretty picture.

10. Notify the patient's physician of an unresponsive poor appetite and ask if any particular drugs could be contributing to the problem.

READY...AIM...APPETITE

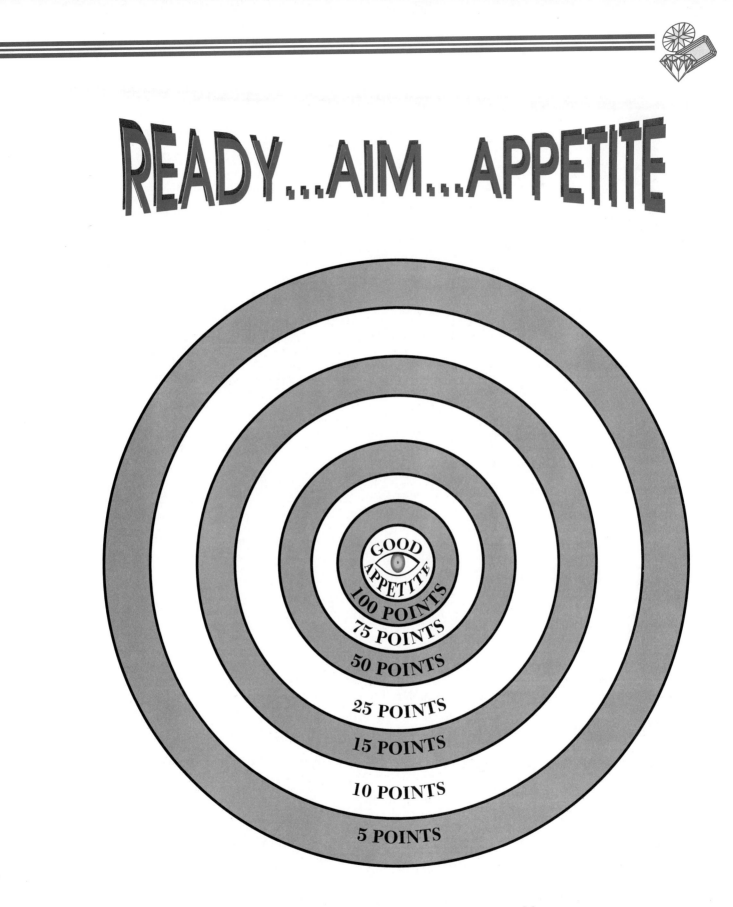

List (in the rings) the steps you are taking to stimulate the patient's appetite.

SQUEAKY CLEAN

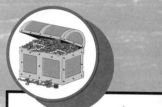

BATHING THE PATIENT (CAREGIVER ROLE)

Treasure Chest

"Making The Most of Bath Time"

"Squeaky Clean"

"Squeaky Clean" answer key

Teaching icon: rubber ducky or squeaky toy (optional) and bar of soap and washcloth

Pen or pencil with an eraser

PREPARATION

1. Copy and review "Making The Most Of Bath Time."
2. Copy "Squeaky Clean."
3. Copy "Squeaky Clean" answer key.
4. Decide on an icon. Suggestions: squeaky toy, rubber ducky, bar of soap, and washcloth.
5. Practice making a bath mitt with the washcloth.
6. Make sure the caregiver has a pen or pencil with an eraser.

IMPLEMENTATION

1. Place the teaching icon in view (i.e., on table) and discuss "Making The Most Of Bath Time" sheet with the caregiver.
2. When finished, have the caregiver complete the "Squeaky Clean" sheet by filling in the bubbles. If the patient is able, encourage participation.
3. Complete the blanks for type of bath and bath frequency according to doctor's orders.
4. Correct any missed answers according to the answer key.
5. Demonstrate making a bath mitt. Have the caregiver make a bath mitt as you discuss bath time and skin care.
6. Leave "Making The Most Of Bath Time" and "Squeaky Clean" with the patient's caregiver.

By: Gaye Ragland, RN, BSN

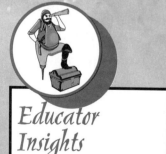

Educator Insights

Be careful not to convey that the patient is not clean. Do convey the importance of well cared-for skin.

MAKING THE MOST OF BATH TIME

· ·

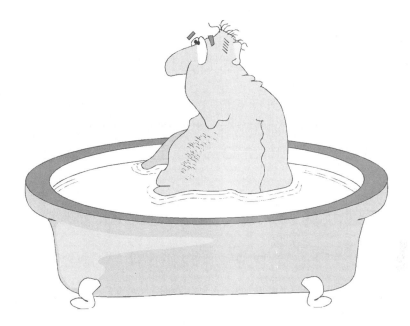

The skin is to the body what armor is to the warrior. The skin serves as a barrier to keep germs out. Therefore, cleansing of the skin is an important part of the daily care of the patient.

Bath time should be a time of comfort and relaxation for the patient. The bath should last no longer than 20 minutes. Make bath time a pleasant experience by following the steps listed below:

◆ Adjust the room temperature of the bathroom. Allow time for the room to reach the desired temperature.

◆ Be sure the room is free of drafts.

◆ Gather all supplies before the bath begins so the patient is not left alone.

◆ Use a rubber mat in the tub to prevent slipping.

29

◆ Fill the tub halfway with water. Do not place the patient in the tub while the water is running. If the water is too hot it may cause a burn.

◆ Check the temperature of the water with your elbow or a bath thermometer. If you use a bath thermometer the water temperature should be 105°F.

◆ DO NOT let the patient check the temperature of the water with his feet. Many patients have a loss of sensation in their feet and could not respond to hot water.

◆ Pull the curtains and close the door for privacy.

◆ Keep the patient covered as much as possible.

◆ Remember, if the patient becomes weak or faints while in the tub, the first thing to do is let out the water.

Now you are ready for the patient to get into the tub. Once the patient is in the tub, wash his body thoroughly. To wash the arm, shoulder, and armpits use long, firm strokes and wash toward the heart. Gently rub the back and shoulders in a circular motion. Unless the patient requests it, do not put soap on the face, since soap is especially drying to the skin. When the soap is not being used, keep it in the soap dish. This prevents the water from becoming excessively soapy, which may cause the patient to become slippery and make it more difficult to thoroughly rinse the patient.

When finished, drain the water. When the water is gone, assist the patient to rise slowly. Pat the skin dry. Do not rub the skin. Keep the patient covered to prevent him from becoming chilled.

And finally, follow specific doctor's orders for bathing frequency. Too frequent baths cause excessively dry skin. Avoid the use of alcohol and deodorant soaps on the skin. These agents tend to overly dry the skin.

TYPE OF BATH ORDERED FOR THE PATIENT:

_____

FREQUENCY OF BATH:

_____

SPECIFIC BATH INSTRUCTIONS:

_____

_____

_____

SQUEAKY CLEAN

DIRECTIONS: Fill in the bubbles.

1. Before the bath begins, adjust the ⬭⬭⬭⬭⬭ ⬭⬭⬭⬭⬭ and eliminate any drafts.

2. Always check the ⬭⬭⬭⬭⬭ of the bath water.

3. Test the water temperature with your ⬭⬭⬭⬭⬭ or with a ⬭⬭⬭⬭⬭ ⬭⬭⬭⬭⬭.

4. Bathtime is the best time to examine the body for ⬭⬭⬭⬭⬭, ⬭⬭⬭⬭⬭, ⬭⬭⬭⬭⬭, etc.

5. Keep the ⬭⬭⬭⬭⬭ out of the water while bathing to prevent the water from becoming too soapy.

6. Because soap tends to dry the skin, do not put soap on the ⬭⬭⬭⬭⬭.

7. If the patient should become weak or faint while in the tub, the first thing to do is let out the ⬭⬭⬭⬭⬭.

8. ⬭⬭⬭⬭⬭ the skin dry.

9. When the bath is finished, have the patient rise ⬭⬭⬭⬭⬭.

10. Keep the body ⬭⬭⬭⬭⬭ as much as possible to prevent the patient from becoming chilled and to provide ⬭⬭⬭⬭⬭.

TYPE OF BATH _____

HOW OFTEN _____

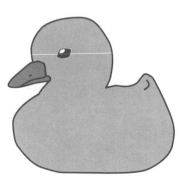

32

SQUEAKY CLEAN

ANSWER KEY:

1. Before the bath begins, adjust the *ROOM TEMPERATURE* and eliminate any drafts.
2. Always check the *TEMPERATURE* of the bath water.
3. Test the water temperature with your *ELBOW* or with a *BATH THERMOMETER*.
4. Bathtime is the best time to examine the body for *BRUISES, CUTS, SORES, ETC.*
5. Keep the *SOAP* out of the water while bathing to prevent the water from becoming too soapy.
6. Because soap tends to dry the skin, do not put soap on the *FACE*.
7. If the patient should become weak or faint while in the tub, the first thing to do is let out the *WATER*.
8. *PAT* the skin dry.
9. When the bath is finished, have the patient rise *SLOWLY*.
10. Keep the body *COVERED* as much as possible to prevent the patient from becoming chilled and to provide *PRIVACY*.

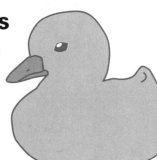

CLEAN AS A WHISTLE

PREPARATION

1. Copy "Clean As A Whistle" crossword puzzle.
2. Copy the answer key to "Clean As A Whistle" crossword puzzle.
3. Make sure the caregiver has a pen or pencil with an eraser.

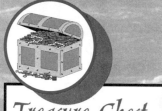

Treasure Chest

"Clean As A Whistle" crossword puzzle

"Clean As A Whistle" crossword puzzle answer key

Pen or pencil with an eraser

IMPLEMENTATION

1. Encourage the caregiver to complete the crossword puzzle.
2. Explain that the answers to the clues may be found in the fact sheet, "Making The Most Of Bath Time."
3. Check the answers to the puzzle when completed or leave the answer sheet (folded together with the answers out of view) and the caregiver may check the answers when the crossword puzzle is completed.
4. Leave "Clean As A Whistle" crossword with the patient's caregiver.

By: Gaye Ragland, RN, BSN

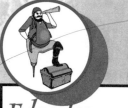

Educator Insights

Remind the caregiver to squat, never stoop, when bending over to run the bath water and when bathing the patient.

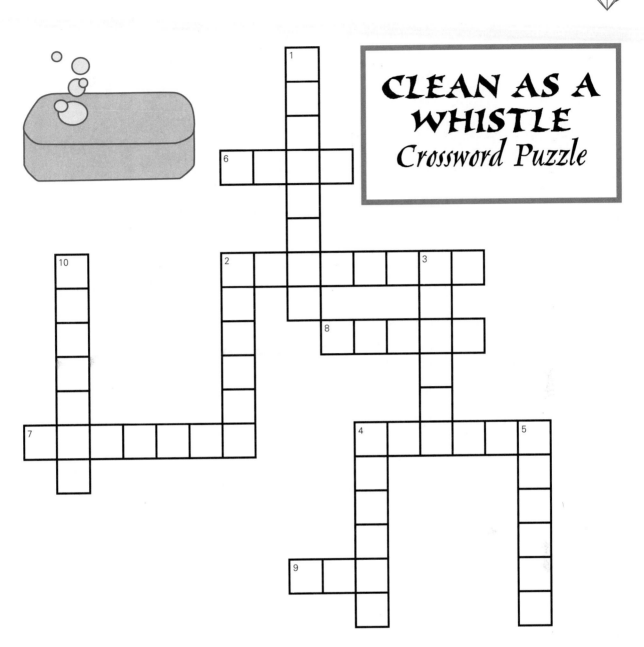

CLEAN AS A WHISTLE
Crossword Puzzle

ACROSS

2. Where the soap is kept when not being used.
4. Soap tends to have a _____ effect on the skin.
6. Because of soap's drying effects, many people prefer no soap on their _____ .
7. Protect the patient's _____ at all times.
8. Check the water temperature with your _____ .
9. How to dry the patient's skin.

DOWN

1. Rub the back and shoulders in a _____ motion.
2. Take steps at bath time to ensure the patient's _____ .
3. When assisting the patient out of the tub, assist the patient to rise _____ .
4. To prevent the patient from becoming chilled, see that the bathroom is free from _____ .
5. _____ all of the needed supplies before the bath begins.
10. A warm bath will promote _____ .

35

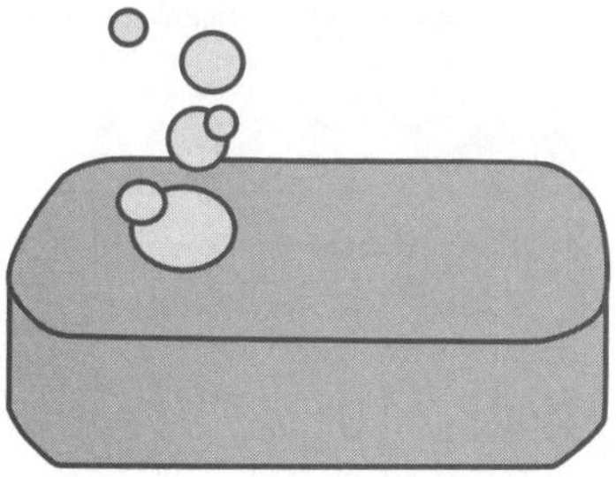

CLEAN AS A WHISTLE
Crossword Puzzle

ANSWER KEY

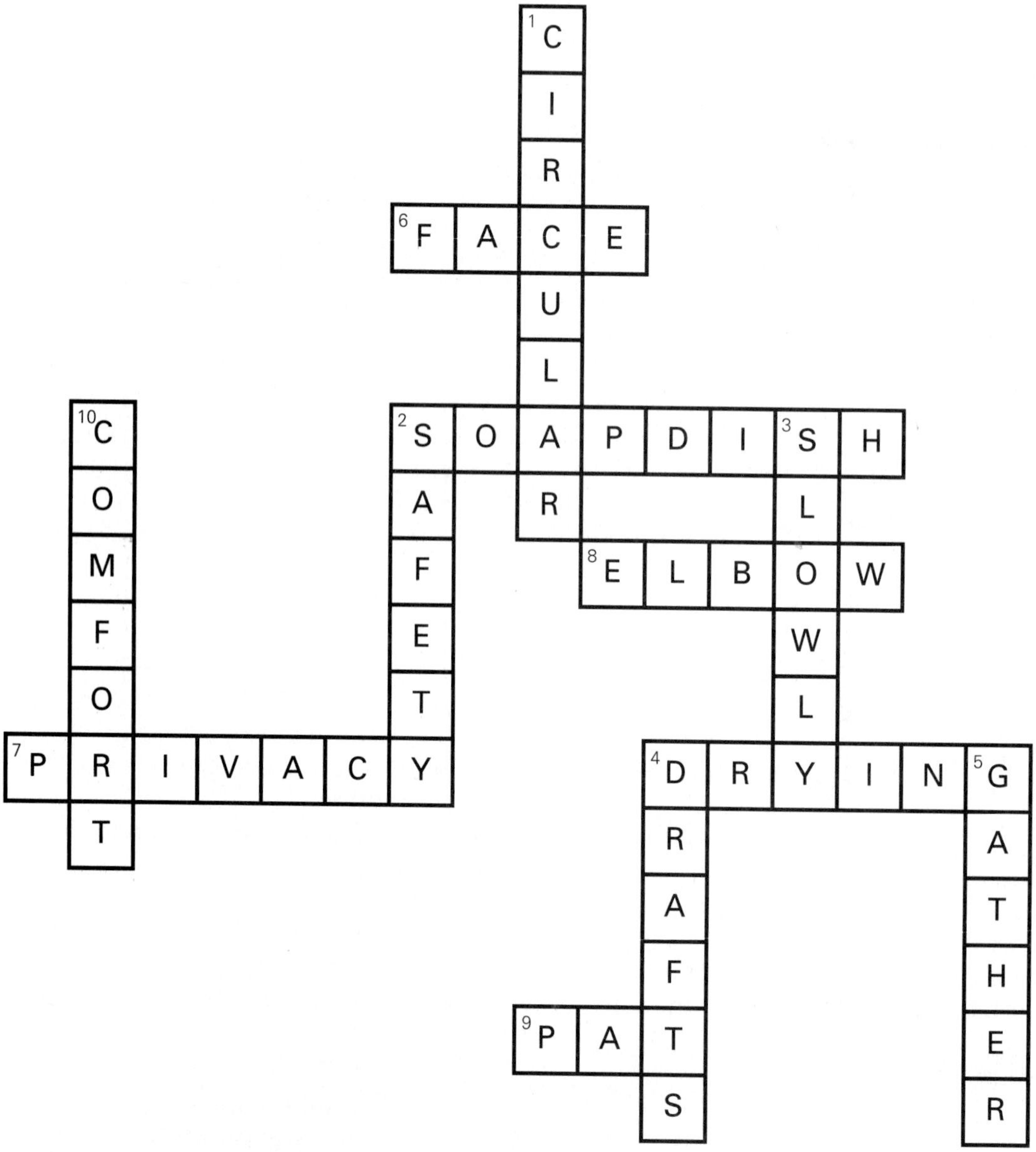
1 CIRCULAR
2 SOAPDISH
3 SLOWL
4 DRYING
4 DRAFTS
5 GATHER
6 FACE
7 PRIVACY
2 SAFETY
8 ELBOW
9 PATS
10 COMFORT

SEARCHING FOR THE SOAP

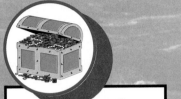

Treasure Chest

"Searching For The Soap"
word search puzzle

"Searching For The Soap"
answer key

Pen or pencil with an
eraser

Educator Insights

Teach the caregiver that
bath time is a good time
to examine the patient's
skin for red areas,
changes in warts or
moles, bruises, cuts, or
abrasions. Notify the
nurse or physician of any
significant changes.

PREPARATION

1. Copy "Searching For The Soap" word search puzzle
   for caregivers.
2. Copy "Searching For The Soap" answer key.
3. Make sure the caregiver has a pen or pencil with an
   eraser.

IMPLEMENTATION

1. Ask the caregiver to complete the word search
   puzzle.
2. Explain that the words hidden in the puzzle are
   items to take into the bathroom at bath time.
3. Check the answers with the caregiver when finished
   or leave the answer sheet folded together with the
   answers out of view and the caregiver may check
   the answers when the word search puzzle is
   completed.

By: Gaye Ragland, RN, BSN

SEARCHING FOR THE SOAP
Word Search

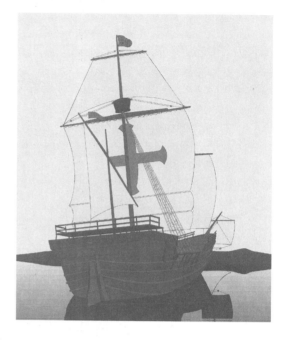

Directions: Circle the hidden items you may take into the bathroom at bath time.

Remember: Words can be forward, backward, up, down, and diagonal.

O	O	P	M	A	H	S	P	Q	H
P	D	A	H	R	C	T	N	E	A
N	O	N	B	B	Z	N	O	T	I
I	R	T	F	J	M	A	I	S	R
G	S	I	S	L	I	P	T	A	B
H	H	E	T	O	I	H	O	P	R
T	I	S	Z	Q	A	B	L	H	U
G	R	B	X	W	Q	P	M	T	S
O	T	A	O	C	E	S	U	O	H
W	P	O	W	D	E	R	D	O	C
N	P	A	J	A	M	A	S	T	B

WORDS

Soap	Shampoo	Slip	Panties
Hairbrush	Toothpaste	Nightgown	Bra
Powder	Housecoat	Comb	Pants
Pajamas	Lotion	Shirt	

38

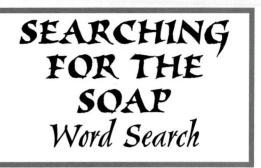

SEARCHING FOR THE SOAP
Word Search

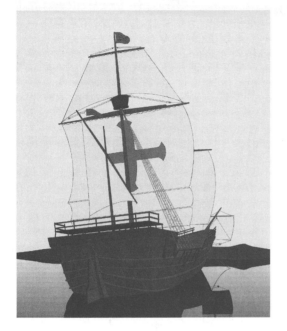

ANSWER KEY:

O	O	P	M	A	H	S	P	Q	H
P	D	A	H	R	C	T	N	E	A
N	O	N	B	B	Z	N	O	T	I
I	R	T	F	J	M	A	I	S	R
G	S	I	S	L	I	P	T	A	B
H	H	E	T	O	I	H	O	P	R
T	I	S	Z	Q	A	B	L	H	U
G	R	B	X	W	Q	P	M	T	S
O	T	A	O	C	E	S	U	O	H
W	P	O	W	D	E	R	D	O	C
N	P	A	J	A	M	A	S	T	B

39

"PEN" THE TAIL (BONE) ON THE SKELETON

Treasure Chest

"Skin Deep"

"'Pen' The Tail (Bone) On The Skeleton"

"Hot Spots To Watch"

Red foil stars
or
Colored sticky dots
or
Red marker

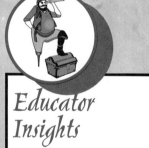

Educator Insights

Alert the caregiver that redness is the first sign of skin breakdown.

PREPARATION

1. Copy and review "Skin Deep" fact sheet.
2. Copy and review "'Pen' The Tail (Bone) On The Skeleton."
3. Copy "Hot Spots To Watch."
4. Identify pressure points throughout the body.
5. Make sure the caregiver has red foil stars, colored sticky dots, or a red marker.

IMPLEMENTATION

1. Review "Skin Deep" fact sheet with the caregiver.
2. Point to "pressure points" on your body and name them one by one.
3. Give the caregiver 30 or so red stars (or red dots or red marker) and instruct the caregiver to mark the pressure points on the pictures on "'Pen' The Tail (Bone) On The Skeleton" that are the areas of greatest risk for skin breakdown.
4. Using "Hot Spots to Watch" as an answer key, complete the diagram by marking any spots missed by the caregiver.
5. Leave "Skin Deep," "'Pen' The Tail (Bone) On The Skeleton," and "Hot Spots To Watch" with patient's caregiver.

By: Gaye Ragland, RN, BSN

SKIN DEEP

Information About Skin Care That Every Caregiver Should Know

Many elderly patients are at risk of forming **pressure ulcers**. It is important that you, as caregiver, know what causes pressure sores and specific measures to prevent their development.

"Pressure ulcer" (better known as a "bedsore" or "skin breakdown"), is a term used to describe tissue destruction in a certain local area of the body. A pressure ulcer is directly related to prolonged **pressure**. There are other contributing factors that cause the bedsore to form. Other factors that can contribute to skin breakdown are: prolonged moisture, poor nutrition, friction, presence of a disease, infection, elevated temperature, or poor circulation.

Remember all risk factors as you care for the patient's skin. Friction occurs when two surfaces rub across one another. When a patient is in the bed a layer of skin tissue can actually be "rubbed" away if the patient is pulled across the linen. This may happen as the patient's position is changed or when the patient's linen is changed. "Shearing" occurs as the patient's skin is stretched until torn. Shearing may occur if a patient sitting up in a bed is allowed to slide down in the bed. As the weight of the patient's body draws him downward, outer tissues that stay in place tend to stick to the bed linen.

As the tissues are being pulled in opposite directions, the result is stretching and ultimately tearing of the tissue. You may not see the tear and the damage to the delicate tissue just under the outer layer of skin. Moisture due to loss of bladder control, wound drainage, or sweating can damage the skin. Patients who are unable to walk or freely move about are at the greatest risk of skin breakdown. It is essential that these patients have their position changed frequently. Patients who cannot turn themselves should be turned every two hours. Wheelchair patients should be repositioned every two hours if they cannot do this for themselves.

Taking steps to provide relief from prolonged pressure is vital to the well-being of the patient. **Pressure points** are common areas of skin breakdown over bony areas. These points must be inspected for signs of redness or irritation. The patient must be turned or lifted and repositioned every two hours. If you notice a reddened area that stays red after ten minutes, this is a warning to you, the caregiver, that the patient must be turned and repositioned more often. Show the reddened area to the nurse. Instruct the patient, if able, to make small shifts of weight as often as possible. Even small movements lessen the risk of skin breakdown.

Bony areas that are potential breakdown sites should be examined as skin care is given. Use lotion for backrubs. It lubricates the skin and lessens the effects of friction or shearing. Do not use rubbing alcohol because it has a drying effect on the skin. Instead, use a lanolin-based moisturizer. Use elbow and heel protectors, along with sheepskins to protect bony prominences. **Pressure reduction** devices such as water mattresses and gel pads are available. Doughnut devices are not recommended. Remember: there is nothing as good for the patient's skin as *good nursing care.*

SPECIAL SKIN CARE INSTRUCTIONS:

_____

_____

_____

_____

_____

_____

_____

_____

_____

_____

"PEN" THE TAIL (BONE) ON THE SKELETON

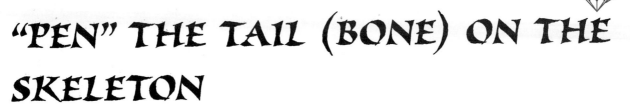

Instructions: Make an "X" on the bony prominences where pressure sores occur most often.

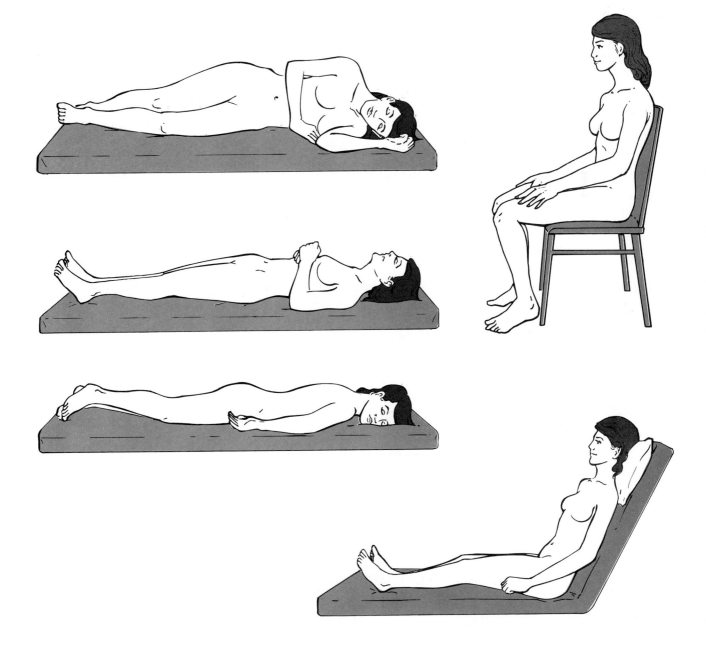

From: *Mosby's Textbook for Nursing Assistants"*, 3rd edition, by Sheila S. Sorrentino, pg. 222.

HOT SPOTS TO WATCH

Answer key: Listed below are the most common pressure ulcer sites:

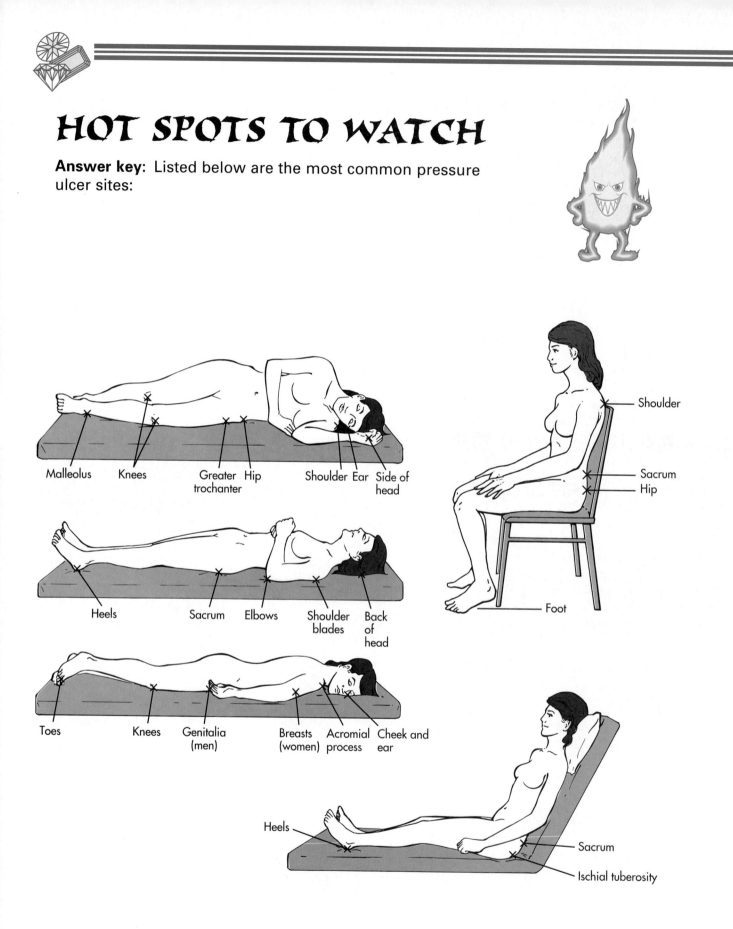

Malleolus   Knees   Greater   Hip   Shoulder   Ear   Side of
                      trochanter   head

Heels   Sacrum   Elbows   Shoulder   Back
                             blades   of
                                         head

Toes   Knees   Genitalia   Breasts   Acromial   Cheek and
                 (men)   (women)   process   ear

Shoulder

Sacrum
Hip

Foot

Heels   Sacrum

Ischial tuberosity

From: *Mosby's Textbook for Nursing Assistants"*, 3rd edition, by Sheila S. Sorrentino, pg. 222.

DON'T MISS THE TURN

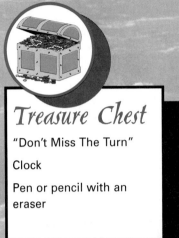

Treasure Chest

"Don't Miss The Turn"

Clock

Pen or pencil with an eraser

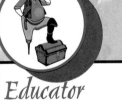

Educator Insights

Amend instructions on record if the patient is restricted from being turned to any particular position.

PREPARATION

1. Copy "Don't Miss The Turn" on one sheet of paper, using both the front and back side of paper.
2. Make sure the caregiver has a pen or pencil with an eraser.

IMPLEMENTATION

1. Explain to the caregiver the directions for completing "Don't Miss The Turn."
2. Start recordkeeping by completing the month (abbreviation) under the word "Date." Explain that the numbers under the word "Date" represent the days of the month.
3. With the caregiver's assistance, decide on a location for turnsheet and pencil that will be close to the patient's bed.
4. Explain that the record will last for one month.
5. Leave "Don't Miss The Turn" with the patient's caregiver.

By: Gaye Ragland, RN, BSN

45

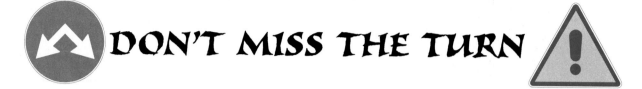

DON'T MISS THE TURN

INSTRUCTIONS: Mark (L) Left, (R) Right, (B) Back, as the patient is turned.

DATE	2 am	4 am	6 am	8 am	10 am	12 noon	2 pm	4 pm	6 pm	8 pm	10 pm	12 mn
1												
2												
3												
4												
5												
6												
7												
8												
9												
10												
11												
12												
13												
14												
15												
16												
17												
18												
19												
20												
21												
22												
23												
24												
25												
26												
27												
28												
29												
30												
31												

46

SQUATTER'S RIGHTS

Treasure Chest

"Squatter's Rights"

"Squatting Right? or Wrong?"

Scissors

Bowl

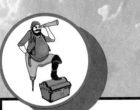

Educator Insights

An empty bathpan is a good prop to use as the "load."

Demonstrate using the patient's wheelchair for rolling a heavy load.

PREPARATION

1. Copy and review "Squatter's Rights."
2. Copy "Squatting Right? or Wrong?"
3. Cut "Squatting Right? or Wrong?" strips, fold and place them in a plastic bag, or you may wait and cut the strips at the teaching site.

IMPLEMENTATION

1. Review "Squatter's Rights" with the caregiver.
2. Put "Squatting Right? or Wrong?" strips in a small bowl.
3. Take turns with the caregiver drawing a strip from the bowl. Follow directions on the strip as body mechanics principles are demonstrated.
4. Leave "Squatter's Rights" with the patient's caregiver.

By: Gaye Ragland, RN, BSN

SQUATTER'S RIGHTS

How To Bend, Lift, and Squat the Right Way

As you provide care for the helpless patient or even for the patient with limited mobility, the lifting and moving, if done incorrectly, can put you at risk for injury. It is important to make the most of the body's strength as you avoid fatigue, strain or injury. By following the RIGHT rules below you will be able to provide care in a safe manner and you may feel less tired at the end of the day.

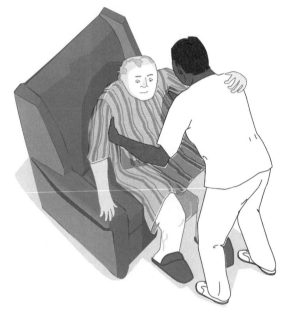

Spread your feet 12" apart before moving a heavy load.

Move close to the load you are about to lift.

Push, pull, or roll a heavy object, rather than lift it.

Use both hands rather than one hand to pick up a piece of heavy equipment.

Use good posture. Keep your back straight and your knees bent.

Always face your work area.

Avoid twisting your body at your waist.

When lifting an object, squat close to the load.

Do not bend (stoop) over from the waist.

Lift by pushing up with the strong, large leg muscles.

If the load is too large or heavy, get help.

If you have help, work together as a team by counting, "1 . . 2 . . 3."

48

SQUATTING

RIGHT? or *WRONG?*

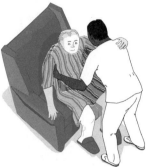

DIRECTIONS: Cut the following rules and activities along the lines. Fold each strip of paper and place them in a small bowl. Taking turns with the caregiver, select an activity from the bowl. Each of you, if possible, demonstrate the instructions on the strips of paper.

Caution: These activities should be attempted only if the caregiver's physical condition allows them to safely perform the demonstration.

DEMONSTRATE SQUATTING AND DESCRIBE HOW YOUR LEG MUSCLES FEEL.
DEMONSTRATE GOOD POSTURE.
DEMONSTRATE BENDING YOUR KNEES.
DEMONSTRATE SQUATTING CLOSE TO THE LOAD.
DEMONSTRATE KEEPING YOUR BACK STRAIGHT WHILE SQUATTING.
DEMONSTRATE GRASPING THE OBJECT FIRMLY.
DEMONSTRATE TURNING WITHOUT TWISTING YOUR BACK.
DEMONSTRATE PIVOTING WITH YOUR FEET.
DEMONSTRATE PUSHING, PULLING, OR ROLLING AN OBJECT RATHER THAN LIFTING IT.
DEMONSTRATE USING BOTH HANDS RATHER THAN ONE.
DEMONSTRATE KEEPING YOUR WEIGHT EVENLY BALANCED ON BOTH FEET.
DEMONSTRATE FACING YOUR WORK AREA.
DEMONSTRATE COUNTING "ONE, TWO, THREE" WITH YOUR PARTNER.
DEMONSTRATE ASKING FOR HELP.
DEMONSTRATE POSITIONING YOUR FEET 12" APART.

PART 3

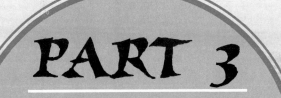

Instant Treasures for Diabetic Teaching

AS THE NEEDLE STICKS

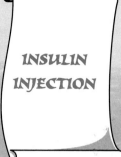

PREPARATION

1. Copy and review "As The Needle Sticks."
2. Determine a comfortable, well-lighted work area.

IMPLEMENTATION

1. Review "As The Needle Sticks" with the patient.
2. Explain the importance of learning self-administration of insulin.
3. Go over each step allowing the patient to practice on the orange until you and the patient feel that the patient is ready to begin self-injecting.
4. Leave "As The Needle Sticks" with the patient.

By: Billie Phillips, MSN, RN

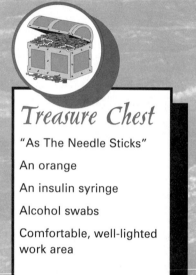

Treasure Chest

"As The Needle Sticks"

An orange

An insulin syringe

Alcohol swabs

Comfortable, well-lighted work area

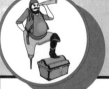

Educator Insights

Remember, the pace at which people learn varies from one individual to the next. Do not rush the patient! This only increases the patient's anxiety.

AS THE NEEDLE STICKS

One Family's Battle with Insulin Administration

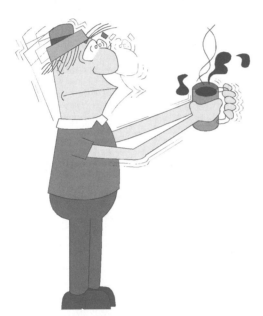

MEET HARRY, WHO HAS A SECRET. HARRY IS AN INSULIN-DEPENDENT DIABETIC WHO TAKES INSULIN SHOTS EVERY DAY.

The Secret! Harry won't give his own insulin shots. It's not that he can't. Harry just won't. So Harry has someone give his shots for him.

MEET EMMA, WHO IS HARRY'S WIFE. EMMA GIVES HARRY HIS INSULIN SHOTS EVERY DAY. EMMA HAS A SECRET WISH.

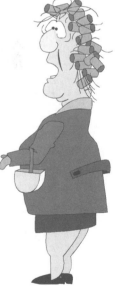

THE SECRET WISH: Emma wishes that Harry would learn to give his own insulin shots. It's not that Emma minds giving them to Harry. But since Harry refuses to learn to give his own shots, and since Harry depends on Emma to always give them for him, Emma is not able to go visit her mother in Tennessee. Emma wishes that Harry would be more independent and responsible in meeting his health care needs. Harry hasn't made any effort to learn to self-administer insulin.

53

MEET SALLY. SHE IS A HOME HEALTH NURSE. LIKE HARRY'S WIFE EMMA, HARRY'S DOCTOR BELIEVES THAT HARRY SHOULD GIVE HIS OWN INSULIN SHOTS. SO HARRY'S DOCTOR HAS ARRANGED FOR SALLY, THE HOME HEALTH NURSE, TO VISIT HARRY.

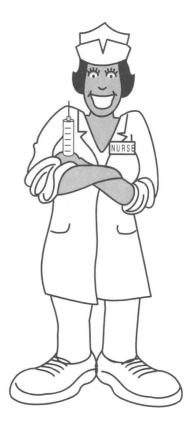

On the first few visits, Harry and Sally talked about diabetes. Then, one day Sally explained to Harry that it was important for him to give his own insulin. At first Harry refused, but Sally continued to explain the importance of self-administration of insulin and was understanding of Harry's feelings. Finally, Harry said he would try.

THE BIG DAY

Sally and Harry sat down at the table with a syringe, a bottle of insulin, alcohol swabs, and an orange. Sally made sure the lighting was good and that Harry was comfortable. Sally explained each step, showing Harry how to draw up the prescribed dose of insulin. Using the orange, she showed Harry how to insert the needle and inject the insulin.

DRAWING THE INSULIN INTO THE SYRINGE

1. Sally explained to Harry that he should wash his hands thoroughly.

2. Next, Sally showed Harry how to roll the insulin bottle gently in his hands.

54

3. Then Sally showed Harry how to use an alcohol swab to clean the top of the insulin bottle.

4. Sally then explained to Harry that he should pull the plunger back to the number of units of insulin to be injected. Even though Harry got a little nervous, he inserted the needle into the bottle and injected the air.

5. Next, Sally showed Harry how to turn the bottle upside-down while withdrawing the prescribed dosage of insulin.

6. Sally explained to Harry to keep the needle under the fluid level, as he checked for air bubbles.

7. Although Harry felt good about drawing up his own insulin, he became very nervous. Sally understood and was very patient and supportive. She explained to Harry that they would proceed slowly and she would continue to explain everything in a step by step manner as she had before.

INJECTING THE INSULIN

1. Sally explained to Harry that he should clean the injection site by swabbing the area with alcohol using a circular motion.

2. Then Sally used an orange to show Harry how to hold the needle at a 45 degree angle and insert the needle into the skin, using a firm deliberate motion. Now she waited patiently for Harry to insert the needle into his skin. Harry was hesitant, so she showed him the procedure again. Slowly but surely HARRY DID IT! Inside, Harry was feeling a great sense of accomplishment, but Harry's face had an expression of "What Do I Do Next?"

3. Sally explained that he should inject the insulin into the tissue by slowly pushing the plunger, and Harry did just that.

4. Harry remembered to gently cover the tip of the needle with an alcohol swab as he withdrew the needle. Harry continued to hold the swab over the site briefly.

NEEDLE DISPOSAL

Sally taught Harry the importance of disposing of the needle in a puncture-resistant container. She explained that he could use a metal/tin container with a lid (suggestion: a metal coffee can with a lid). She taught Harry to empty the container when it is half full. She also told Harry never to push the used syringes into the opening of the used needle container. They talked about how infections can be passed through needlesticks. She explained how important it was to keep the container out of the reach of children.

Sally waved goodbye to Harry and said she would be back the next day. She came every day for one week until she was sure that Harry was comfortable with the technique of giving his own insulin. Three weeks later when she stopped by, Harry invited her into the house. He said he was glad to see her. Emma was in Tennessee with her mother.

MEET HARRY, WHO IS AN INSULIN-DEPENDENT DIABETIC, BUT IS NOW INDEPENDENT WHEN IT COMES TO GIVING HIS INSULIN SHOTS.

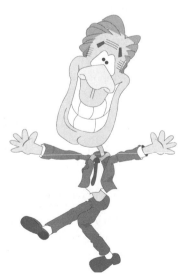

TIC-TAC-"TOE"

PREPARATION

1. Review "'Tic-Tac-Toe' Foot Care Facts" game pieces.
2. Make two copies of "'Tic-Tac-Toe' Foot Care Facts" game pieces.
3. Copy "Tic-Tac-Toe" game board.
4. Cut game pieces along lines so that each "Foot Care Facts" game piece is cut apart separately. You may choose to cut paper strips at the teaching site.
5. Put paper strips in a small sandwich bag.
6. Make sure the caregiver has a pen or pencil with an eraser.

IMPLEMENTATION

1. Fold each of the "Foot Care Facts" game pieces.
2. Place all 22 folded facts into a small bowl. Play 4 games of "Tic-Tac-Toe" with the patient after deciding who will be player "X" and who will be player "O."
3. Before each player makes a mark, the player must draw a "Foot Care Fact" and read it aloud to the other.
4. If the patient is unable to read, the nurse will read a fact before each mark is made.
5. Use the shoe icon as a visual aid as foot care is taught.
6. When finished, explain that the winner is the one who practices daily foot care.
7. Leave "'Tic-Tac-Toe' Foot Care Facts" with the patient.

By: Gaye Ragland, RN, BSN

Treasure Chest

"'TIC-TAC-TOE' Foot Care Facts"

"TIC-TAC-TOE" game pieces sheet

Old shoe as a visual icon

Pen or pencil with an eraser

Educator Insights

An old worn out shoe is a good visual aid to use as proper foot care is taught. Be sure to stress the importance of proper footwear.

TIC-TAC-TOE
Foot Care Facts

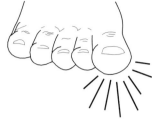

Directions: Cut Foot Care Facts along the lines. Fold each strip of paper and place them in a small bowl. Draw in turn and read the fact. Then take a turn at **"TIC-TAC-TOE"** Foot Care Facts.

WASH YOUR FEET DAILY.
WASH YOUR FEET WITH LUKEWARM WATER AND SOAP.
DRY YOUR FEET WELL.
ALWAYS DRY BETWEEN THE TOES.
USE AN EMERY BOARD TO SHAPE YOUR TOENAILS.
SHAPE YOUR TOENAILS EVEN WITH THE END OF YOUR TOES.
KEEP THE SKIN OF YOUR FEET SUPPLE (FLEXIBLE).
USE A MOISTURIZING LOTION, BUT NOT BETWEEN THE TOES.
CHANGE DAILY INTO SOFT SOCKS OR STOCKINGS.
ONLY WEAR SHOES THAT FIT.
SHOES THAT DO NOT FIT MAY RUB BLISTERS.
KEEP YOUR FEET WARM.
KEEP YOUR FEET DRY.
WEAR PADDED SOCKS.
WEAR LEATHER SHOES.
DO NOT WALK BAREFOOTED.
DO NOT WEAR SOCKS OR STOCKINGS THAT ARE TOO BIG.
EXAMINE YOUR SHOES FOR CRACKS OR ROUGH EDGES.
INSPECT YOUR FEET DAILY.
WHEN INSPECTING YOUR FEET, LOOK BETWEEN THE TOES.
WATCH FOR REDNESS, PAIN, NUMBNESS, OR WOUNDS.
NOTICE AND REPORT ANY WOUNDS (SORES) THAT DO NOT HEAL.

58

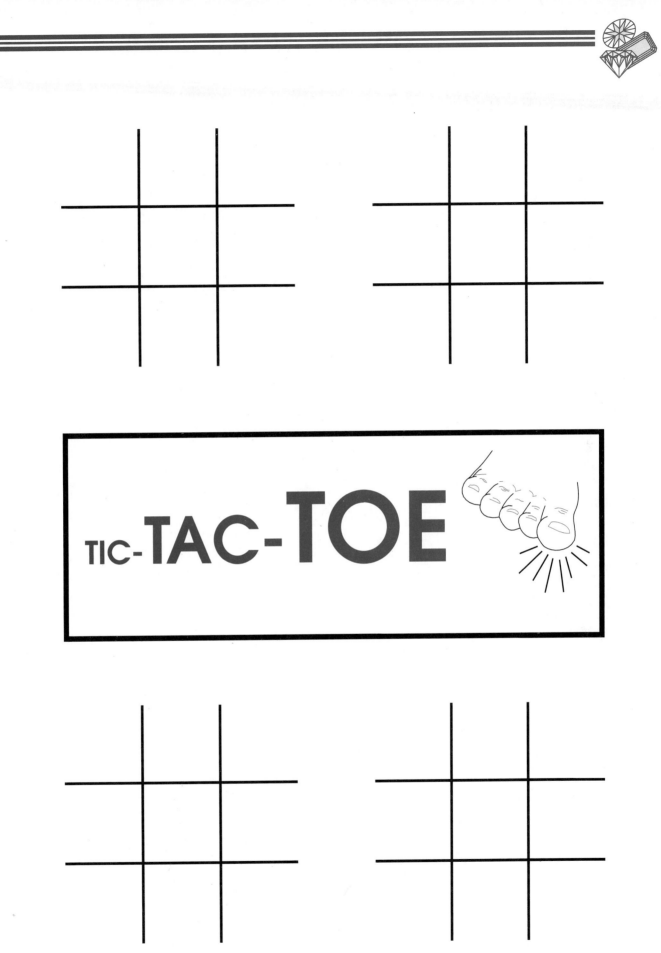

TIC-TAC-TOE

NEVER OUT OF SITE(s)

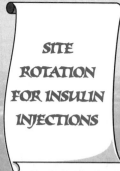

SITE ROTATION FOR INSULIN INJECTIONS

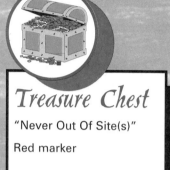

Treasure Chest

"Never Out Of Site(s)"

Red marker

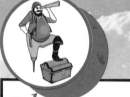

Educator Insights

Indicate the proper areas on the body for site for insulin rotation by marking them on the body picture.

PREPARATION

1. Copy and review "Never Out of Site(s)."
2. Make sure the patient has a red marker.

IMPLEMENTATION

1. Discuss proper rotation of sites for insulin injections using "Never Out Of Site(s)."
2. With the red marker, make dotted lines around suggested areas for insulin injection.
3. Have the patient indicate the areas on the body being presently used for injections.
4. Leave "Never Out of Site(s)" with the patient.

By: Susan Lofton, RN, MSN

Never Out of Site(s)

WHAT KIND OF SITES?

Sites for insulin injection.

WHAT ABOUT THE SITES?

Rotate insulin sites.

WHY SHOULD I ROTATE MY INSULIN SITES?

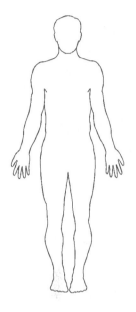

Rotating insulin sites helps reduce the likelihood of infection and skin damage. Otherwise, you may experience a buildup of scar tissue and lumpy skin areas which are unsightly and damaging to your body. Also, if you use one area repeatedly, this causes the insulin to be administered into scar tissue. This in turn causes your insulin to be poorly absorbed in this one area.

WHERE ARE THE SITES I SHOULD USE?

ARMS—the outer part of your upper arms.

STOMACH—just above and below your waist, but do avoid the tender area around your navel.

BACK—on both sides, below your waist, just above your hip bones.

THIGHS—front and outsides of both thighs.

HOW SHOULD I ROTATE?

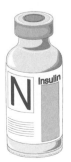

Inject into one area for about one week. Don't put the needle into the exact same spot, but use the same general area for one week (example - upper right arm).

Rotate to a different site area each week. Choosing a specific weekday for site change is a good idea. You may decide that every Sunday will be "new site day."

ON THE ROAD AGAIN

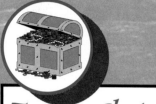

Treasure Chest

"On The Road Again"

Travel magazine or brochure

Blunt scissors

Tape

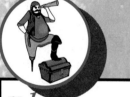

Educator Insights

Travel agencies will often provide free brochures loaded with travel pictures.

PREPARATION

1. Copy and review "On The Road Again."
2. Be sure caregiver has a travel magazine or brochure, blunt scissors, and tape.

IMPLEMENTATION

1. Look at the travel brochure. Talk about places the patient has been as well as places the patient would like to go.
2. Using "On The Road Again," discuss travel tips for the diabetic.
3. You may assist the patient with preparing the list of medical information suggested to be carried "On The Road Again."
4. Leave "On The Road Again" with the patient.

By: Susan Lofton, RN, MSN

....ON THE ROAD AGAIN....

Notes for the Diabetic Traveler

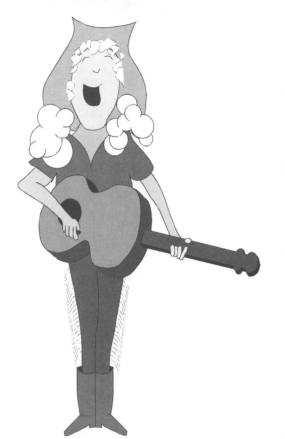

- Check with your doctor before taking long or extended trips. Your doctor may wish to see you for a checkup before you go.
- Pack enough insulin, syringes, and all other necessary medical supplies to last the duration of the trip. Then pack a few extra.
- Make a list of all your current medications, the exact amount and type of insulin you are taking, the diet you are following, and the name and phone number of your physician, pharmacist, and nearest relative at home. Keep this list in your wallet or purse for quick access in case of an emergency. Ask a traveling companion to keep a copy of your list, as well.
- Be sure your traveling companion(s) know that you are a diabetic. Discuss the symptoms of hypo- and hyperglycemia with them. Be sure your companions know where a convenient supply of quick glucose (sugar) is located, and where you keep your daily supply of insulin. As you pack, remember to pack a bag to keep with you containing those items that you may need quickly.

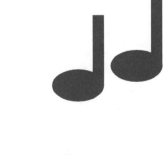

- If traveling by plane, tell your travel agent that you are a diabetic. Airlines will supply diabetic snacks or meals if notified ahead of flight time. Be sure to closely monitor your blood sugar level. Changes in diet and activity levels can cause sudden changes in your blood sugar levels.
- Be sure to provide plenty of rest intervals for yourself.
- Have fun!

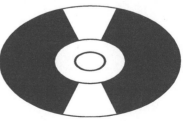

63

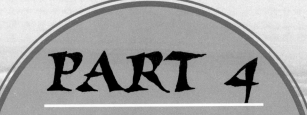

PART 4

Instant Treasures for Diet Teaching

SODIUM SURVEY

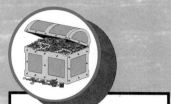

Treasure Chest

"Straight Talk About Sodium"

"Sodium Survey"

Pen or pencil with an eraser

PREPARATION

1. Review "Straight Talk About Sodium."
2. Review and copy "Sodium Survey."
3. Make sure the patient has a pen or pencil with an eraser.

IMPLEMENTATION

1. Review "Sodium Survey" with the patient.
2. Read the directions to the patient.
3. Assist the patient, if necessary, to check the answers in the appropriate column.
4. Analyze the survey with the patient to determine those high-sodium foods most frequently eaten.
5. Leave "Sodium Survey" with the patient.

By: Gaye Ragland, RN, BSN

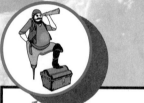

Educator Insights

This tool also works well for the patient with limited reading skills. You read the questions aloud and check the correct column as the patient verbalizes the answers. The patient can then be shown the number of check marks on the right side of the page, indicating the high amount of sodium intake.

Straight Talk About Sodium

Table salt is the main source of sodium in the diet. We absorb nearly all of the sodium that we eat and this well absorbed mineral becomes a key factor in the retaining of body water.

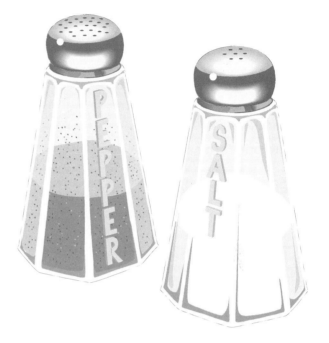

If we ate only fresh foods (not packaged or canned) without adding salt, we would take in the minimum recommended daily allowance of about 500 mg of sodium a day. However, the average adult usually gets from about 3000 to 7000 mg a day by eating processed foods and by adding salt as food is cooked. From one-third to one-half of the sodium we get is added as food is cooked or once the food makes it to the table. Most of the rest of the salt is added during food manufacturing.

Some people are what is said to be "sodium-sensitive." If you have high blood pressure, the doctor has probably instructed you to reduce the amount of salt you eat. In addition to high blood pressure, if you have problems with your heart, liver, or kidneys, your doctor may have placed you on a "reduced sodium" diet.

As you begin to work at reducing the amount of sodium in your diet, you should first examine your own pantry. Find those foods you are presently eating that should either be eaten in moderation or completely removed from your shelves.

It is also important to know that your nurse, doctor, or dietician will give you some suggestions for foods that can be used for flavoring in the place of salt. Also, most people who are placed on a low-sodium diet do adjust. At first you may feel that the food has no flavor. Some patients say that the food is "bland." However, most patients do adjust to this new way of eating and are soon able to regulate their sodium intake to the level prescribed by their doctor.

Sodium Survey

Directions: Answer the following questions about the foods you eat and how you prepare them. The more answers you have in the columns to the right, the higher your sodium intake.

	Less than One Time a Week	1 to 2 Times a Week	3 to 5 Times a Week	Almost Daily
1. Eat popcorn				
2. Eat canned soup?				
3. Drink tomato juice?				
4. Eat potato chips?				
5. Eat peanuts?				
6. Eat luncheon meat or canned meat?				
7. Eat weiners, bacon, sausage, or ham?				
8. Eat frozen boxed prepared meals?				
9. Add sauces to foods like catsup, steak sauce, soy sauce, etc.?				
10. Eat pickles?				
11. Add salt to water when cooking vegetables, rice, or pasta?				
12. Add bacon or pork to vegetables?				
13. Add seasoning salts to foods?				
14. Add salt to your food once it is on the table?				
15. Add broth (canned or cubes) to your food?				
20. Add salt to your food before you ever taste it?				

SODIUM SCAVENGER HUNT

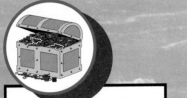

Treasure Chest

"Sodium Scavenger Hunt"

"Sodium Scavenger Hunt Suggestions for Substitutes"

Pen or pencil with an eraser

Educator Insights

Looking through the patient's pantry should be done only with permission from the patient. Always remember, you are a guest in the patient's home (or room).

PREPARATION

1. Review and copy "Sodium Scavenger Hunt."
2. Read "Sodium Scavenger Hunt Suggestions for Substitutions" before starting the activity.
3. Make sure the patient has a pen or pencil with an eraser.

IMPLEMENTATION

1. Review "Sodium Scavenger Hunt" directions with the patient.
2. Identify high-sodium foods that are in the patient's pantry and list them on the "Sodium Scavenger Hunt".
3. Teach the patient to read labels.
4. For each high-sodium food found, suggest a lower sodium substitute that is in compliance with the patient's prescribed diet and list it on the "Sodium Scavenger Hunt".
5. Leave "Sodium Scavenger Hunt" with the patient.

By: Gaye Ragland, RN

SODIUM SCAVENGER HUNT

Directions: With the patient's assistance, search the pantry and refrigerator for foods with high sodium content. In the left column list the high sodium foods. In the right column, list a suggested "low-sodium" substitute.

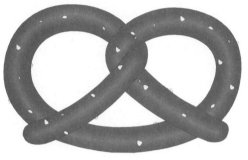

High-Sodium Food   **Suggested Substitute**

_____

_____

_____

_____

_____

_____

_____

_____

_____

_____

NOTES: _____

_____

_____

_____

SODIUM SCAVENGER HUNT

*Suggestions for Substitutes**

*Suggested substitutes are acceptable only in accordance with prescribed diet.

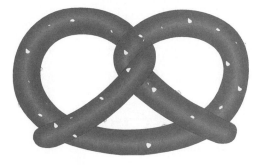

High Sodium Food	Suggested Substitute
Salt	Herbs and spices
Canned, cured meats Cold cuts	Fresh meats
Regular crackers	Low salt crackers
Popcorn	Unsalted popcorn
Seasoning salt	Seasoning powder
Buttermilk	Whole, lowfat, or skim milk (up to 2 cups a day) (Low sodium milk if specified by doctor)
Canned soups	Homemade soups with no salt added or canned soup with no salt added
Canned vegetables	Fresh vegetables with no salt added
Nuts, pretzels	Unsalted nuts, unsalted pretzels
Salted snacks in general	Fresh fruits

READ FOOD LABELS CAREFULLY. WATCH FOR WORDS LIKE SALT AND SODIUM IN THE LIST OF INGREDIENTS.

TOMATO-BASED FOODS IN GENERAL TEND TO BE HIGH IN SODIUM.

71

SEARCHING FOR THE SODIUM

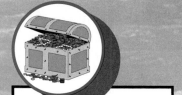

SODIUM RESTRICTED DIET

PREPARATION

1. Copy "Searching For The Sodium" word search puzzle for the patient.
2. Copy the answer key for "Searching For The Sodium."
3. Make sure the patient has a pen or pencil with an eraser.

IMPLEMENTATION

1. Ask the patient to complete the word search puzzle.
2. Explain that the words hidden in the puzzle are high-sodium foods.
3. Check the answers with the patient's answers when finished or leave the answer sheet (folded together with the answers out of view). The patient may check the answers whenever the word search puzzle is completed.
4. Leave "Searching For The Sodium" with the patient.

By: Gaye Ragland, RN, BSN

Treasure Chest

"Searching For The Sodium"

"Searching For The Sodium" answer key

Pen or pencil with an eraser

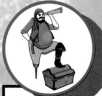

Educator Insights

Remind the patient that the words can go up and down, backward, forward, etc.

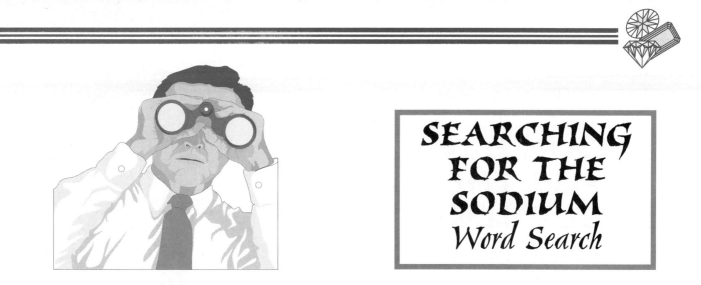

SEARCHING FOR THE SODIUM
Word Search

Directions: Search the puzzle for the foods that have a high amount of sodium.*

Remember: Words can be forward, backward, up and down, and diagonal.

P	T	C	O	L	D	C	U	T	S
I	L	C	H	I	P	S	H	A	M
C	A	A	S	A	L	T	S	T	O
K	S	O	Y	S	A	U	C	E	L
L	O	C	P	N	B	N	Y	N	I
E	N	M	U	S	T	A	R	D	V
S	A	U	S	A	G	E	Z	Y	E
Z	J	T	T	E	N	P	U	O	S
P	O	T	A	T	O	C	H	I	P
T	Q	O	C	H	E	E	S	E	E
S	O	U	P	Z	B	A	C	O	N
M	I	L	K	O	Q	N	T	L	Z

WORDS:

Ham	Sausage	Potato Chip	Pickles
Chips	Cheese	Salt	Milk
Soy Sauce	Cold Cuts	Salt	Olives
Peanuts	Mustard	Soup	Bacon

This puzzle references regular, not "low salt" or "no salt" version foods.

73

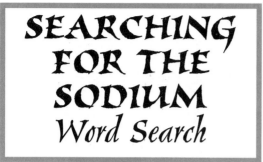

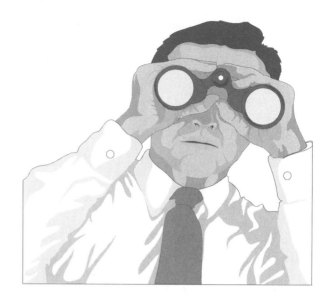

ANSWER KEY:

P	T	C	O	L	D	C	U	T	S	S
I	L	C	H	I	P	S	H	A	M
C	A	A	S	A	L	T	S	T	O
K	S	O	Y	S	A	U	C	E	L
L	O	C	P	N	B	N	Y	N	I
E	N	M	U	S	T	A	R	D	V
S	A	U	S	A	G	E	Z	Y	E
Z	J	T	T	E	N	P	U	O	S
P	O	T	A	T	O	C	H	I	P
T	Q	O	C	H	E	E	S	E	E
S	O	U	P	Z	B	A	C	O	N
M	I	L	K	O	Q	N	T	L	Z

74

SOOO SALTY

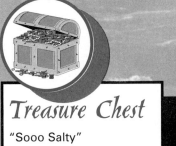

Treasure Chest

"Sooo Salty"

"Sooo Salty" answer key

Pen or pencil with an eraser

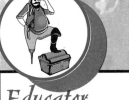

Educator Insights

To further reduce sodium, suggest draining and rinsing canned vegetables prior to cooking.

PREPARATION

1. Copy "Sooo Salty" word search puzzle for the patient.
2. Copy the answer key for "Sooo Salty."
3. Make sure the patient has a pen or pencil with an eraser.

IMPLEMENTATION

1. Ask the patient to complete the word search puzzle.
2. Explain that the words hidden in the puzzle are the names of high sodium foods.
3. Check the answers with the patient when finished or leave the answer sheet (folded together with the answers out of view). The patient may check the answers when the word search puzzle is complete.
4. Leave "Sooo Salty" puzzle with the patient.

By: Gaye Ragland, RN, BSN

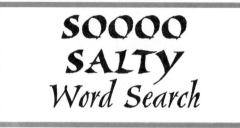

SOOOO SALTY
Word Search

Directions: Find the hidden foods that are "Soooooo Salty"*:

P	S	T	E	A	K	S	A	U	C	E	K	T	J
O	L	I	V	E	S	N	U	T	S	V	R	L	O
T	C	Y	B	R	O	T	H	H	D	B	O	A	S
A	O	U	S	T	U	N	O	C	A	B	P	S	R
T	L	H	E	P	P	I	C	K	L	E	S	E
O	D	S	E	N	I	D	R	A	S	Q	C	O	N
C	C	C	O	R	N	C	H	I	P	S	F	Y	E
H	U	N	C	R	A	C	K	E	R	S	I	S	I
I	T	N	R	O	C	P	O	P	T	F	B	A	W
P	S	Y	O	J	A	K	W	C	A	T	S	U	P
S	O	D	A	Z	N	L	E	S	E	E	H	C	M
S	A	L	T	S	H	A	K	E	R	K	G	E	X

HOW MANY DID YOU FIND?

WORDS:

Potato Chips   Olives   Corn Chips   Catsup
Cold Cuts   Nuts   Crackers   Wieners
Soup In A Can   Broth   Salt Shaker   Salt
Soy Sauce   Pickles   Soda   Pork
Steak Sauce

*This puzzle references regular, not low salt or no salt version foods

76

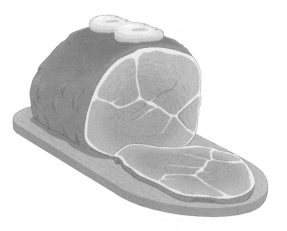

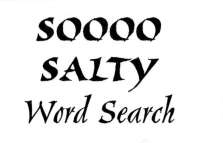

SOOOO SALTY
Word Search

ANSWER KEY:

P	S	T	E	A	K	S	A	U	C	E	K	T	J
O	L	I	V	E	S	N	U	T	S	V	R	L	O
T	C	Y	B	R	O	T	H	H	D	B	O	A	S
A	O	U	S	T	U	N	O	C	A	B	P	S	R
T	L	H	E	P	P	I	C	K	L	E	S	E	
O	D	S	E	N	I	D	R	A	S	Q	C	O	N
C	C	C	O	R	N	C	H	I	P	S	F	Y	E
H	U	N	C	R	A	C	K	E	R	S	I	S	I
I	T	N	R	O	C	P	O	P	T	F	B	A	W
P	S	Y	O	J	A	K	W	C	A	T	S	U	P
S	O	D	A	Z	N	L	E	S	E	E	H	C	M
S	A	L	T	S	H	A	K	E	R	K	G	E	X

DID YOU FIND ALL 17?

77

FIND THE FAT (FOODS)

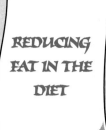

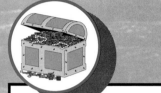

Treasure Chest

"Find The Fat" word search puzzle

"Find The Fat" answer key

Pen or pencil with an eraser

PREPARATION

1. Copy "Find The Fat" word search puzzle.
2. Copy the answer key for "Find The Fat" word search puzzle.
3. Make sure the patient has a pen or pencil with an eraser.

IMPLEMENTATION

1. Ask the patient to complete the word search puzzle.
2. Explain that the words hidden in the puzzle are foods especially high in fat content.
3. Check the answers with the patient when finished or leave the answer sheet (folded together with the answers out of view). The patient may check the answers whenever the word search puzzle is completed.
4. Leave "Find The Fat" with the patient.

By: Gaye Ragland, RN, BSN

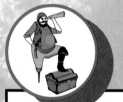

Educator Insights

As the patient identifies favorite foods that are high fat, suggest lower fat substitutes that are good tasting and nutritious.

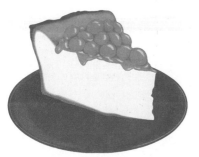

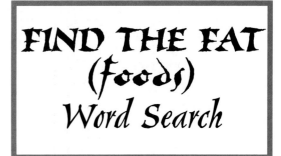

FIND THE FAT (foods) Word Search

The fat in some foods is easy to see. Name some types of food fats that are easy to spot.

Other foods are loaded with fat, but the fat is not so obvious. Try to name some foods that have large amounts of hidden fat.

Buried in the box below are foods that have a high fat content. Search the box and **"Find the Fat" foods.** Can you find all 12?

REMEMBER: Words can be forward, backward, up and down, and diagonal.

B	U	T	T	E	R	S	O	L	O
A	M	A	E	R	C	E	C	I	D
V	T	T	I	M	B	S	S	L	O
O	E	L	P	V	O	I	S	E	U
C	H	O	C	O	L	A	T	E	G
A	U	K	R	R	O	N	U	S	H
D	S	U	E	A	G	N	N	E	N
O	A	N	A	G	N	O	L	E	U
S	M	O	M	L	A	Y	A	H	T
P	E	A	N	U	T	A	W	C	Z
B	U	T	T	E	R	M	E	U	U

WORDS:

Pie	Cheese	Avocado	Mayonnaise
Peanut Butter	Walnuts	Chocolate	Bologna
Doughnut	Cream	Ice Cream	Butter

79

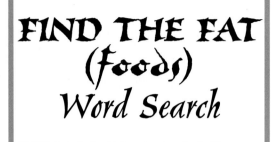

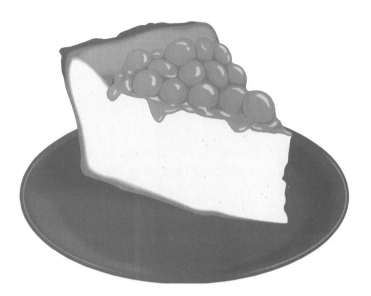

ANSWER KEY:

B	U	T	T	E	R	S	O	L	O
A	M	A	E	R	C	E	C	I	D
V	T	T	I	M	B	S	S	L	O
O	E	L	P	V	O	I	S	E	U
C	H	O	C	O	L	A	T	E	G
A	U	K	R	R	O	N	U	S	H
D	S	U	E	A	G	N	N	E	N
O	A	N	A	G	N	O	L	E	U
S	M	O	M	L	A	Y	A	H	T
P	E	A	N	U	T	A	W	C	Z
B	U	T	T	E	R	M	E	U	U

80

SPOILED ROTTEN

PREPARATION

1. Review and copy "Spoiled Rotten."
2. Review and copy "How To Keep Your Food Physically Fit."
3. Remove 4 to 6 clean labels from food, especially from perishable items.
4. Obtain one can of any type food.

IMPLEMENTATION

1. Place canned food within patient's view.
2. Ask the patient what comes to mind when hearing the saying, "SPOILED ROTTEN."
3. Initiate discussion of safe food handling using "Spoiled Rotten."
4. Offer suggestions for proper food handling using "How To Keep Your Food Physically Fit."
5. Examine food labels as you discuss storage and cooking times according to the labels.
6. Remind the patient to call the grocer if unsure of the proper cooking requirements or shelf/refrigerator life.
7. Remind the patient never to taste food that is suspected to be spoiled.
8. Leave "Spoiled Rotten" and "How To Keep Your Food Physically Fit" with the patient.

By: Gaye Ragland, RN, BSN

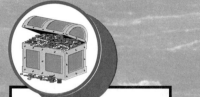

Treasure Chest

"Spoiled Rotten"

"How To Keep Your Food Physically Fit"

4 to 6 clean labels removed from uncooked foods

1 can of food (any type)

Educator Insights

Be careful that your tone is instructional, never critical. "Cleanliness" can be a "touchy" issue.

SPOILED ROTTEN

Food poisoning affects 7 million Americans each year. It causes people to miss work and school and can be quite serious, especially for the very young, very old, or for the patient who is already ill. It is important to take steps to prevent food poisoning, also known as "foodborne illness."

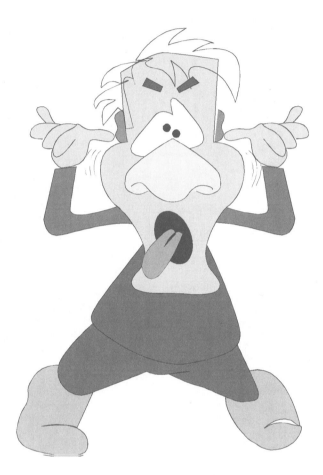

Most germs that cause food poisoning are killed when food is cooked. But when food stays *warm* for 2 hours or more, germs can produce poisons that are not killed by heating the food. In addition, germs cannot reproduce as fast if the food is stored at temperatures *below 40 degrees Fahrenheit.* Though the germs may be busy at work, they usually do not change the ways the food looks, smells, or tastes.

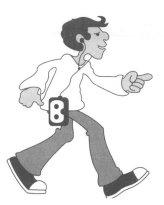

How To Keep Your Food
PHYSICALLY FIT

REMEMBER:

1. Read food labels so you will know how to prepare the food. Some foods are already fully cooked. Others must be cooked before eaten.

2. Keep food hot until it is served.

3. Refrigerate leftover food at once.

4. Cook poultry products thoroughly. If poultry is prepared in advance of cooking, store it in the refrigerator until time for cooking. Do not put stuffing in the bird until you are ready to cook it. Store giblets and stuffing separately.

5. When shopping, pick up meat, poultry, and dairy products last and take them straight home to be refrigerated quickly.

6. The refrigerator life of most meats varies from one to seven days. The meats that will spoil the quickest are ground beef, veal, lamb, ground pork, and variety meats. Smoked sausage, bacon, a smoked whole ham, and corned beef will keep for 7 days.

7. The best way to thaw frozen meat is to place it in the refrigerator during the day or overnight, the night before you intend to cook the meat.

8. Store sandwich meat and wieners in the refrigerator.

9. Do not buy food if the packaging, seals, or lids appear to be damaged or tampered with in any way.

10. Handle meat with forks or tongs. Fingers are a good method for spreading germs.

11. Clean dishes, utensils, serving platters, countertops, and fingers with soap and hot water. Germs live all around us. When preparing food, we must keep the working area and our hands as clean as possible.

12. Do not place cooked meat on the same platter that contained raw meat.

13. Do not place any other food on a cutting board used for raw meat until the board is thoroughly washed with hot water.

14. Keep any sores covered before handling food. Do not handle food at all if you have infected wounds of any kind.

SLIMMING DOWN THE AMOUNT OF SUGAR

CALORIE RESTRICTED DIET

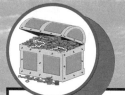

Treasure Chest

"Slimming Down The Amount Of Sugar"

"Names of Sugars Used in Foods"

3 labels from pre-packaged sugar-containing foods

A piece of fruit of your choice

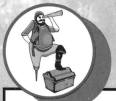

Educator Insights

Using the fruit as a visual icon, explain both the financial as well as the nutritional value of eating healthy.

PREPARATION

1. Review and copy "Slimming Down The Amount Of Sugar."
2. Select three food labels that demonstrate sugar content.
3. Choose a piece of fruit for a visual icon (patient's diet permitting).

IMPLEMENTATION

1. Discuss "Suggestions For Reducing Sugar Intake" and "Names Of Sugars Used In Foods" with the patient.
2. Review the labels of at least three prepackaged sugar-containing foods from the patient's pantry or labels from your "Treasure Chest".
3. Highlight three of the suggestions the patient chooses from the list to be priority attempts for reducing sugar intake.
4. Reward the patient's commitment to healthier eating with a piece of fruit (diet permitting).
5. Leave "Slimming Down The Amount Of Sugar" with the patient.

By: Gaye Ragland, RN, BSN

Slimming Down the Amount of Sugar

SUGGESTIONS FOR REDUCING SUGAR INTAKE*

At the Supermarket
- Read ingredient labels. Identify all the added sugars in a product. Select items lower in total sugar when possible.
- Buy fresh fruits or fruits packed in water, juice, or light syrup, rather than those in heavy syrup.
- Buy fewer foods that are high in sugar, such as prepared baked goods, candies, sweet desserts, soft drinks, and fruit-flavored punches and soft drinks. Substitute vanilla wafers, graham crackers, bagels, English muffins, and diet soft drinks, for example.
- Buy nuts (dry roasted), sunflower seeds, and popcorn (use hot-air popper) to replace candy for snacks.

In the Kitchen
- Reduce the sugar in foods prepared at home. Try new recipes or adjust your own. Start by reducing the sugar gradually until you've decreased it by one third or more.
- Experiment with such spices as cinnamon, cardamom, coriander, nutmeg, ginger, and mace to enhance the flavor of foods.
- Use home-prepared items (with less sugar) instead of commercially prepared ones that are higher in sugar, when possible.

At the Table
- Use less of all sugars. This includes white and brown sugar, honey, molasses, and syrups.
- Choose fewer foods high in sugar, such as prepared baked goods, candies, and sweet desserts.
- Reach for fresh fruit instead of a sweet for dessert or when you want a snack.
- Add less sugar to foods—coffee, tea, cereal, or fruit. Get used to using half as much, then see whether you can cut back even more.
- Cut back on the number of sugared soft drinks and fruit punches you drink. Substitute water, fruit juice, or diet soft drinks.

From the USDA Home and Garden Bulletin No. 232-5, 1986.

NAMES OF "SUGARS" USED IN FOODS:

Sugar

Sucrose

Brown sugar

Confectioner's sugar (powdered sugar)

Turbinado sugar

Invert sugar

Glucose

Levulose

Lactose

Honey

Corn syrup or sweeteners

High fructose corn syrup

Molasses

Maple syrup

Dextrose

Maltose

POTASSIUM IN THE PANTRY

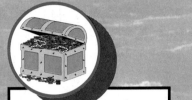

POTASSIUM-RICH FOODS

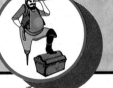

Treasure Chest

"Putting Potassium In Its Place" fact sheet

"Potassium In The Pantry" game sheet

Banana, orange, or sweet potato

Pen or pencil with an eraser

Educator Insights

Fresh meats are higher in potassium than canned or cured; fresh fruits are higher in potassium than canned.

PREPARATION

1. Copy and review, "Putting Potassium In Its Place" fact sheet.
2. Copy "Potassium In The Pantry" game sheet.
3. Make sure the caregiver has a pen or pencil with an eraser.

IMPLEMENTATION

1. Review "Putting Potassium In Its Place" fact sheet with patient.
2. Go over the list of high potassium foods.
3. With the patient's permission and assistance, search the pantry (and refrigerator) for available food sources rich in potassium.
4. Complete the "Potassium In The Pantry" game sheet by listing high potassium foods on hand on the left, and suggestions of several high potassium foods for the patient to purchase on the right.
5. Under "need to buy" column, only list those foods that are acceptable on the patient's prescribed diet. Also, list only those foods that the patient likes, can chew, and can afford.
6. Leave "Potassium In The Pantry" and "Putting Potassium In Its Place" with the patient.

By: Gaye Ragland, RN, BSN

Putting Potassium in its Place

Information About Potassium in the Diet

Most adults get enough potassium in the diet if a broad variety of foods are eaten. However, because as a rule we do not add potassium to the foods we eat (unlike salt) we are more likely to become potassium deficient than we are to become sodium deficient. And then there can be the effect of certain diuretics, better known as "fluid pills." People who take "potassium-wasting" diuretics should have their potassium level checked regularly.

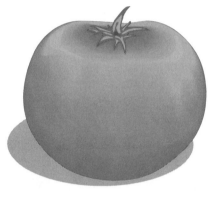

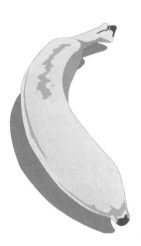

Milk, whole grains, dried beans, and meats are good sources of potassium. Generally, fruits and vegetables are good sources as well. Other foods and fluids that contribute potassium to the diet are coffee, tea, orange juice, potatoes, and milk.

Below is a list of potassium-rich foods. Check with your doctor or nurse for more information to meet your specific dietary needs.

Foods High in Potassium Content

Apricots	Nuts
Artichokes	Oranges, Orange juice
Avocado	Peanuts
Banana	Potatoes
Cantaloupe	Prune juice
Carrots	Pumpkin
Cauliflower	Spinach
Chocolate	Swiss chard
Dried beans, Peas	Sweet potatoes
Dried fruit	Tomatoes, Tomato juice, Tomato sauce
Mushrooms	Watermelon

88

POTASSIUM IN THE PANTRY

HAVE ON HAND	NEED TO BUY

CALCIUM IN THE CABINET

(and fridge, too)

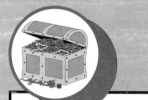

Treasure Chest

"Calcium In The Cabinet" fact sheet

"Calcium In The Cabinet" game sheet

"Good Sources of Calcium" list

Pen or pencil with an eraser

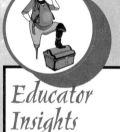

Educator Insights

Milk and dairy products are the only calcium sources some patients can name. Make them aware of others.

PREPARATION

1. Copy and review "Calcium In The Cabinet" fact sheet.
2. Copy and review "Good Sources of Calcium" list.
3. Copy "Calcium In The Cabinet" game sheet.
4. Make sure the patient has a pen or pencil with an eraser.

IMPLEMENTATION

1. Review and discuss "Calcium In The Cabinet" fact sheet with the patient and/or caregiver.
2. Have the patient or the caregiver complete the "Calcium In The Cabinet" game sheet by listing the high calcium foods the patient has on hand as well as suggestions of high calcium foods to buy.
3. Be sure any suggested high calcium foods are within the limits of the diet prescribed by the patient's physician.
4. Leave "Calcium In The Cabinet" fact and game sheets and "Good Sources of Calcium" list with the patient.

By: Nancy Hollis, MSN, RN

Calcium in the Cabinet (and Fridge, Too)

Calcium is an essential mineral to our diets. The body's requirement for calcium varies depending on age and whether we are male or female. But whether we are male or female and regardless of age, calcium is the main source of building material for our bones and teeth. The majority of our calcium is stored in the bones. A small amount of calcium is stored in our teeth. The rest is used to regulate muscles, help our blood clot and to carry signals to and from our brain.

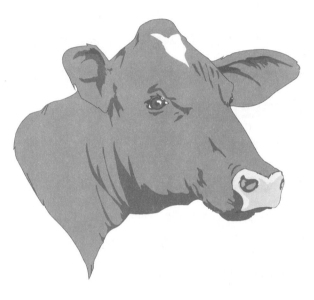

Calcium can be found in milk and yogurt, cheese, selected milk products, broccoli, beet greens, kale, dried lentils, peas, beans, sesame seeds, small fish (sardines) eaten with the bones, clams, and oysters.

An increase in nervousness, muscle spasms or cramps, an irregular heartbeat, or trouble going to sleep are some of the problems that may occur when the body does not have enough calcium. Other problems sometimes seen in patients without enough calcium stored is stunted growth, weak bones, or even convulsions.

The following page lists foods that are high in calcium.

91

GOOD SOURCES OF CALCIUM

✓ MILK

✓ YOGURT

✓ CHEESE

✓ SELECTED MILK PRODUCTS

✓ BROCCOLI

✓ BEET GREENS

✓ KALE

✓ CITRUS FRUITS

✓ DRIED PEAS

✓ DRIED BEANS

✓ SESAME SEEDS

✓ CLAMS

✓ OYSTERS

✓ SMALL FISH (SARDINES) EATEN WITH THE BONES

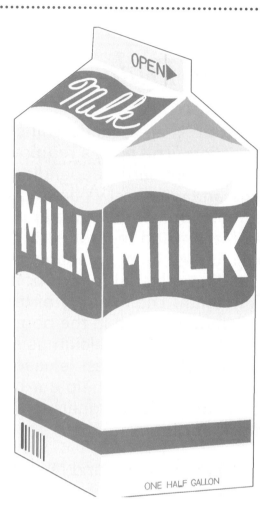

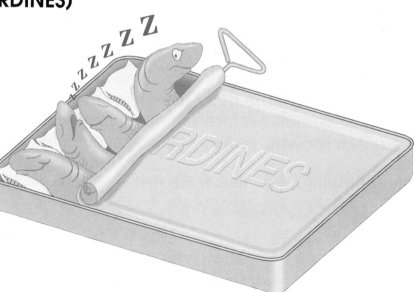

92

CALCIUM IN THE CABINET
(and fridge, too)

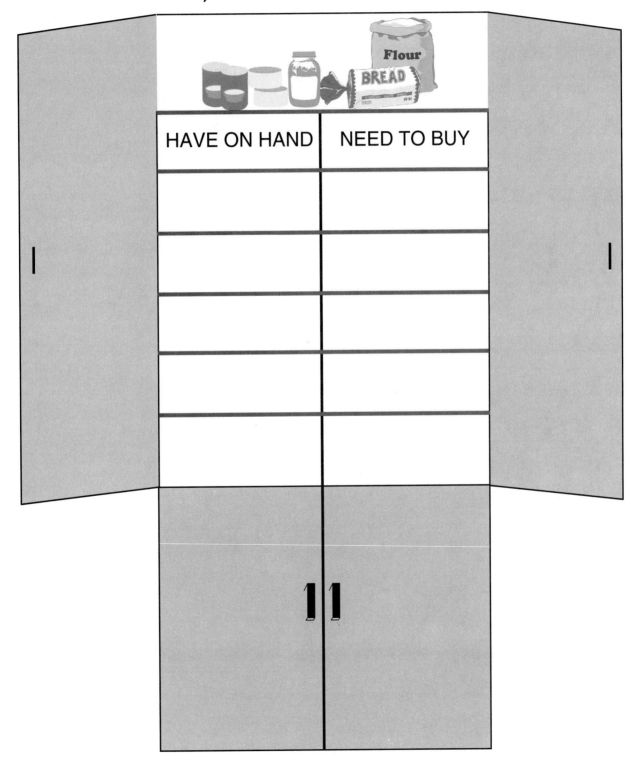

HAVE ON HAND	NEED TO BUY

WHO WANTS A GREASY GLASS?

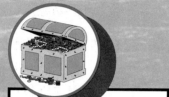

Treasure Chest

"Considering Cholesterol"

A clean drinking glass

Clean water

One teaspoon of cooking oil

Spoon for stirring

One drop of red food coloring

PREPARATION

1. Review "Considering Cholesterol."
2. Obtain a small bottle of red food coloring and seal it in a plastic bag for transporting.

IMPLEMENTATION

1. Ask the patient for a small glass of water, a spoon, and one teaspoon of cooking oil.
2. Add oil and one drop of red food coloring to the glass of water. If the patient is able allow him/her to do the experiment.
3. Stir and discuss how the fat is unable to dissolve into the water. Equate the *red* water to the patient's *red* blood.
4. Have the patient feel the inside of the glass. Talk about the greasy build-up.
5. Move into diet instruction for lowering dietary cholesterol.

By: Gaye Ragland, RN, BSN

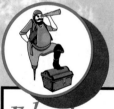

Educator Insights

Be sure to clean up the mess!

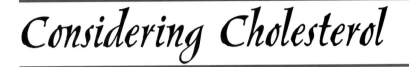

Considering Cholesterol

Inside the body cells is a soft, fat-like substance called cholesterol. Cholesterol is used to make certain hormones in our body. It is also used to make bile which is made in the liver and then stored in the gallbladder. Bile is needed to help us digest the foods we eat. Cholesterol is also used to form cell membranes and other needed tissue.

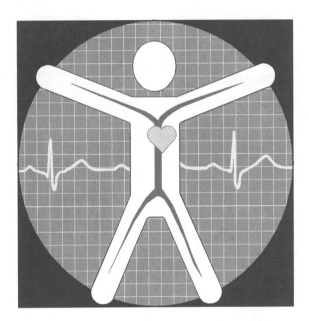

The body gets cholesterol in the following ways: the body makes cholesterol "as needed" and we get cholesterol from certain foods we eat. If our body needs more cholesterol than the amount we eat, the liver manufactures more cholesterol on an "as needed" basis.

The cholesterol that we get from our diet comes from foods that come from animals. Foods that come from plants do not contain cholesterol.

Cholesterol and other fats cannot dissolve in the blood, just like a teaspoon of vegetable oil will not dissolve in a glass of water. Having too much cholesterol in the circulating blood can lead to the build-up of cholesterol in the walls of the arteries that feed the heart and brain. Along with other substances, these deposits build up inside the vessels, similar to rust and corrosion building up inside an old pipe. Eventually, the build-up can clog the vessels, and sometimes the site of this "clogging" is where a blood clot will form. If the clot forms in the heart this results in a heart attack. If the clot forms in the brain, the result is a stroke.

According to the American Heart Association, the desirable range for blood cholesterol is less than 200 mg/dl. From 200 to 239 mg/dl is considered borderline high for total cholesterol. A cholesterol level of 240 mg/dl and over is considered high.

It is important to periodically have your cholesterol checked. Then discuss the findings and the recommendations with your doctor.

WHERE'S THE FAT

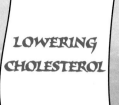

LOWERING CHOLESTEROL

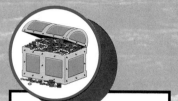

Treasure Chest

"Where's The Fat" quiz

"Where's The Fat" answer key

Pen or pencil with an eraser

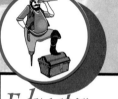

Educator Insights

Have the patient do a self survey. Have the patient identify which food is eaten rarely, occasionally, or frequently.

PREPARATION

1. Review and copy "Where's The Fat" quiz.
2. Copy "Where's The Fat" answer key.
3. Make sure the patient has a pen or pencil with an eraser.

IMPLEMENTATION

1. Ask the patient to complete the cholesterol quiz.
2. Explain that the patient is to look over the list and decide which food (standard serving amount) is the highest in cholesterol. Beside that food write number one. Then find the food with the next highest amount. Then the next and so on until the foods are rated one through twelve.
3. When finished rating the foods, compare the patient's answer to the answer key. Point out which foods are the highest, but explain that all the foods on the sheet are high in cholesterol.
4. Leave "Where's The Fat" with the patient.

By: Gaye Ragland, RN, BSN

"WHERE'S THE FAT?"

Directions: Rate the following foods from **the most (1) to the least (12)** in order of the amount of

CHOLESTEROL

you believe each contains per serving.

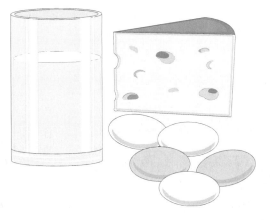

_____ OYSTERS

_____ EGG YOLK

_____ SHRIMP

_____ LARD

_____ WHOLE MILK

_____ MAYONNAISE

_____ LIVER

_____ KIDNEY

_____ HALF AND HALF

_____ HOT DOG

_____ SKIM MILK

_____ CHEDDAR CHEESE

"WHERE'S THE FAT?"

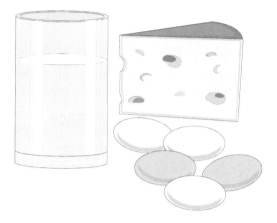

ANSWER KEY:

_5_	OYSTERS		_2_	LIVER
_3_	EGG YOLK		_1_	KIDNEY
_4_	SHRIMP		_9_	HALF AND HALF
_10_	LARD		_8_	HOT DOG
_6_	WHOLE MILK		_12_	SKIM MILK
_11_	MAYONNAISE		_7_	CHEDDAR CHEESE

SCRAMBLED EGGS

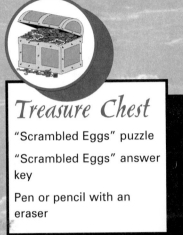

Treasure Chest

"Scrambled Eggs" puzzle

"Scrambled Eggs" answer key

Pen or pencil with an eraser

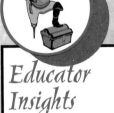

Educator Insights

Have the patient identify frequently eaten "high cholesterol" foods.

PREPARATION

1. Review and copy "Scrambled Eggs" puzzle.
2. Copy "Scrambled Eggs" answer sheet.
3. Make sure the patient has a pen or pencil with an eraser.

IMPLEMENTATION

1. Ask the patient to complete the word scramble puzzle.
2. Explain that the scrambled words are names of high cholesterol foods.
3. Check the patient's answers when finished or leave the answer sheet (folded together with the answers out of view). The patient may check the answers whenever the word scramble puzzle is completed.
4. Leave "Scrambled Eggs" with the patient.

By: Gaye Ragland, RN, BSN

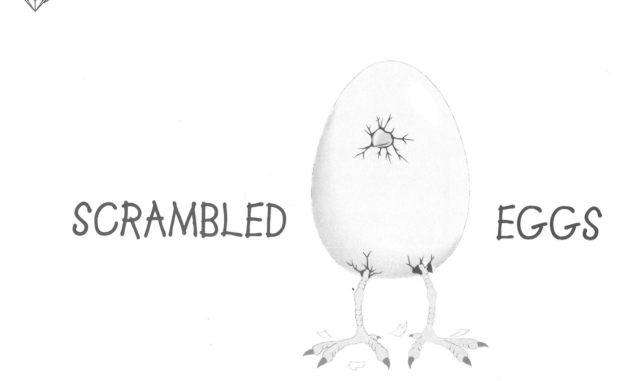

SCRAMBLED EGGS

Directions: Unscramble the following words that raise the blood cholesterol.

ABRSNI   _____

PIMHRS   _____

BETSORL   _____

GEG LOYK   _____

HELOW KIML   _____

RIVLE   _____

RUBTET   _____

DARL   _____

MECAR   _____

NOOTUCC   _____

SCRAMBLED 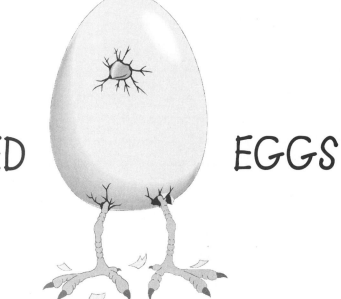 EGGS

ANSWER KEY:

ABRSNI	BRAINS
PIMHRS	SHRIMP
BETSORL	LOBSTER
GEG LOYK	EGG YOLK
HELOW KIML	WHOLE MILK
RIVLE	LIVER
RUBTET	BUTTER
DARL	LARD
MECAR	CREAM
NOOTUCC	COCONUT

I'M READY TO ORDER NOW

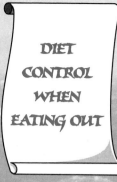

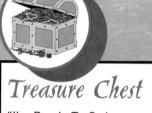

Treasure Chest

"I'm Ready To Order Now"

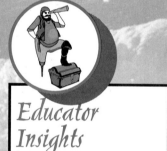

Educator Insights

You and the patient call the patient's favorite restaurant and ask if the restaurant will prepare foods for special diets.

PREPARATION

1. Review and copy "I'm Ready To Order Now."

IMPLEMENTATION

1. Discuss with the patient the tips found on "I'm Ready To Order Now."
2. Consider the special dietary needs of the particular patient with whom you are working. Give the patient ideas of good choices that would be within the patient's prescribed dietary guidelines.
3. Leave "I'm Ready To Order Now" with the patient.

By: Gaye Ragland, RN, BSN

I'm Ready To Order Now

Just because you have special dietary needs doesn't mean you can't eat out. Below are a few tips to remember when eating in a restaurant.

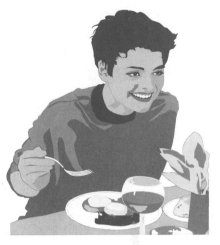

✓ Call ahead and ask about menu choices.

✓ If eating in a crowded dining room causes you to become anxious or to feel rushed, call ahead to determine the restaurant's busiest time. Then make reservations ahead of the crowd.

✓ Ask about specials that are not on the menu.

✓ Ask how the foods are prepared.

✓ Do not hesitate to ask for special preparation for a particular food. For example, if you prefer your entrée broiled rather than fried, ask for it.

✓ If you feel uncomfortable eating in public places because of physical limitations, consider calling ahead to reserve seating in a private dining area of the restaurant. If it is difficult for you to cut your meat, ask that it be cut in the kitchen.

✓ Ask for fat to be trimmed and skin to be removed from foods before they are cooked.

103

✓ Ask for sauces, gravies and dressings to come on the side instead of on the entrée. In doing so, you have control over the amount that is added.

✓ When necessary, ask about substitutions. The menus of some restaurants say "no substitutions." However, if your diet doesn't permit a certain food that comes with an entrée, you may be able to substitute something as simple as a single vegetable or piece of fruit in its place.

✓ If you are on a salt restricted diet, choose a food that can be cooked by itself with no added salt. Be sure to ask that the food be prepared with no salt added.

✓ Ask for margarine instead of butter.

✓ If you are eating eggs, ask about egg substitutes.

✓ If drinking milk with the meal, ask for skim or 1%. If you are drinking coffee or tea, ask about decaffeinated.

. . .ENJOY

MAGAZINE MEAL PLANNING

PREPARATION

1. Tape four pieces of paper together on the back side: two pieces on top and two pieces on bottom to form a large square, slightly smaller than a standard sheet of poster board.
2. Obtain several magazines. Inexpensive women's magazines found at grocery store checkout lines are often loaded with food pictures.

IMPLEMENTATION

1. Look through the magazines with the patient for pictures of foods as you talk about healthy food choices.
2. You and the patient clip out pictures of good choices within the patient's prescribed diet and attach the pictures to the paper in a collage fashion with clear tape.
3. Suggest posting the collage on the refrigerator door as a reminder of healthy eating.
4. You may attach pictures of unacceptable foods and encircle them with bright red ring and "X".

By: Gaye Ragland, RN, BSN

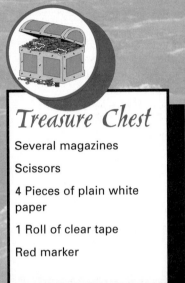

Treasure Chest

Several magazines

Scissors

4 Pieces of plain white paper

1 Roll of clear tape

Red marker

Educator Insights

This exercise is good for teaching diets to the educationally challenged.

DAILY DINER

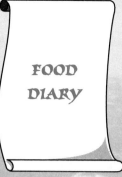

FOOD DIARY

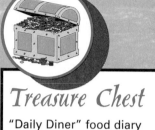

Treasure Chest

"Daily Diner" food diary

Pen or pencil with an eraser

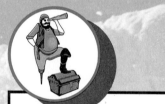

Educator Insights

To conserve paper, make copies of the "Daily Diner" on the front and back side of each sheet.

PREPARATION

1. Copy one "Daily Diner" for every day a food diary is to be kept.
2. Label in advance each sheet with the day of the week it is to be completed.
3. Make sure the patient/caregiver has a pen or pencil with an eraser.

IMPLEMENTATION

1. Explain to the patient how to record all food and drink on the "Daily Diner."
2. Recommend that the patient write the intake as he eats. Recalling the entire day's intake is difficult at the end of the day.
3. Agree upon a safe, convenient place for the copies to be stored until the next visit.
4. Encourage the patient to keep a daily food diary.

By: Gaye Ragland, RN, BSN

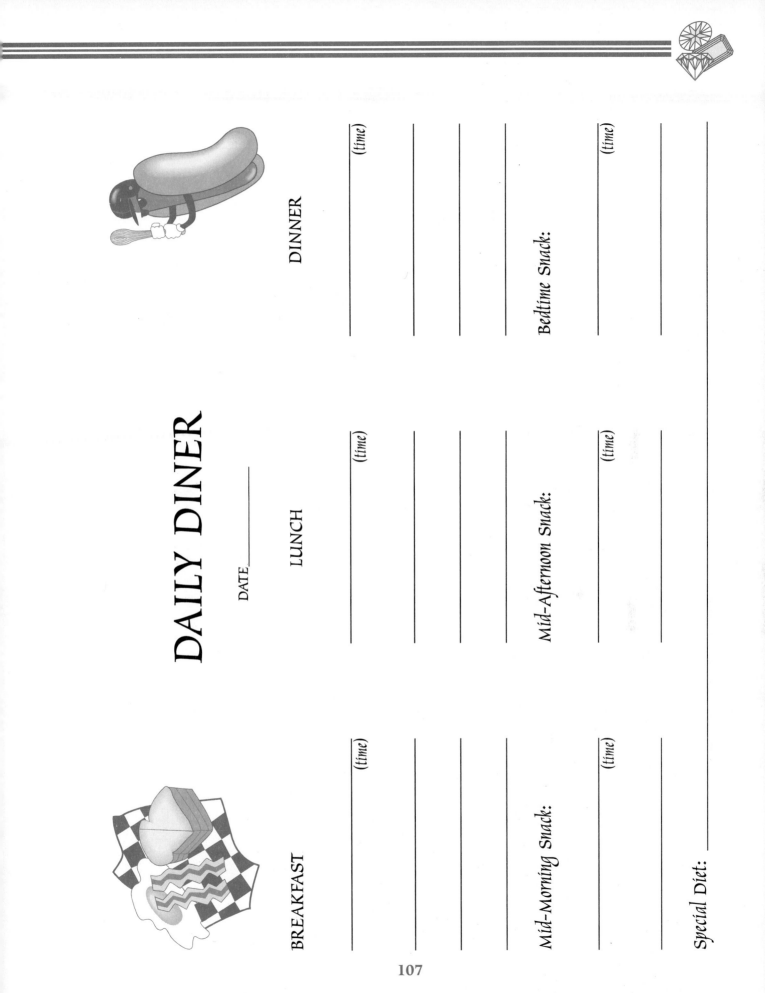

DAILY DINER

DATE_____

BREAKFAST _____(time)

LUNCH _____(time)

DINNER _____(time)

Mid-Morning Snack: _____(time)

Mid-Afternoon Snack: _____(time)

Bedtime Snack:

Special Diet:

107

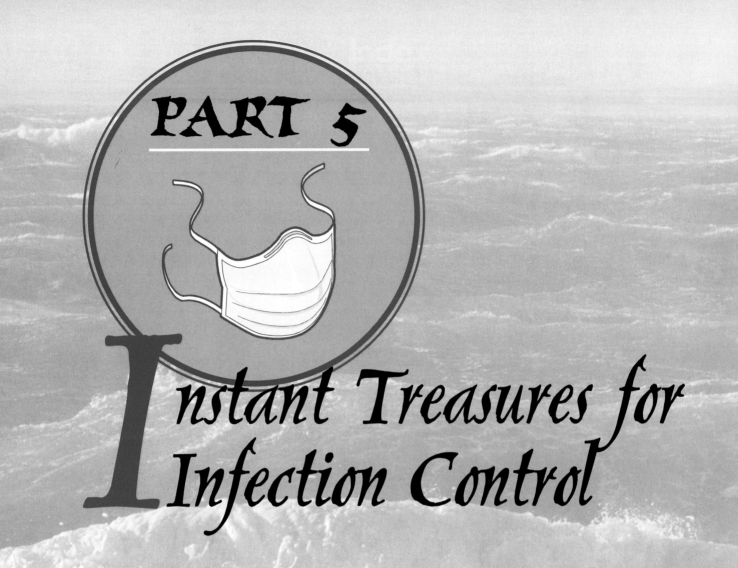

PART 5

Instant Treasures for Infection Control

HANDWASHING TO NEW HEIGHTS

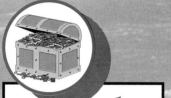

Treasure Chest

"Handwashing to New Heights" fact sheet

"Handwashing To New Heights" game sheet

Access to running water

Bar soap

Orange stick or nail file

Paper towel

Clean towel

Hand lotion

Pen or pencil with an eraser

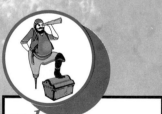

Educator Insights

Stop during the procedure and have the patient or caregiver correct any mistake. Then give credit during the game.

PREPARATION

1. Copy and review "Handwashing To New Heights" fact sheet.
2. Copy and review "Handwashing To New Heights" game sheet.
3. Make sure the patient has soap, a clean towel, and a pen or pencil with an eraser.

IMPLEMENTATION

1. Review and discuss "Handwashing To New Heights" fact sheet with the patient and/or caregiver.
2. Demonstrate proper handwashing techniques after the fact sheet is discussed.
3. Have the patient or caregiver return demonstrate proper handwashing.
4. Circle each step on the "Handwashing To New Heights" game sheet.
5. Leave the "Handwashing To New Heights" fact sheet and game sheet with the patient/caregiver.

By: Gaye Ragland, RN, BSN

HANDWASHING TO NEW HEIGHTS

The easiest and most important way to fight the spread of infection is to wash your hands. Your hands are used in almost everything you do. If handwashing is not practiced properly and frequently, germs causing infection can be easily spread. The following HANDWASHING TIPS should be practiced every day. Your doctor or nurse will tell you of any special soap or additional instructions, if necessary.

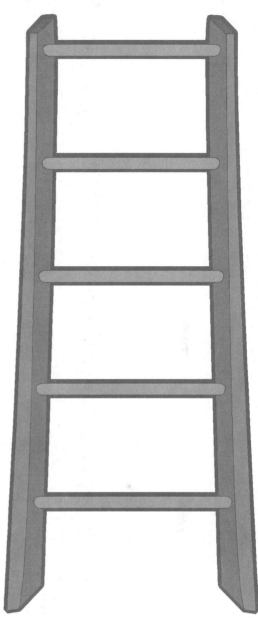

1. Turn on warm, running water. Do not touch the inside of the sink as you wash.

2. Rinse the bar of soap before you use it.

3. Hold the bar of soap during the entire time you are washing your hands.

4. Wet your hands and wrists thoroughly under the running water. Keep your hands lower than your elbows.

5. Use enough soap to work up a good lather. Continue to add water to the soap while you wash.

6. Using friction (rubbing), give special attention to the thumbs, sides of the fingers, knuckles, sides of the hands, and under the fingernails. Use an orange stick or nail file to clean under the fingernails.

7. Continue to wash for 1 to 2 minutes, starting at the fingertips and working toward the forearm.

8. When finished, rinse the soap and drop it into the soapdish. Do not touch the soapdish, since it is contaminated.

9. Rinse your hands well, keeping your fingers pointed downward.

10. Dry your hands and wrists with a clean towel.

11. Using a clean paper towel, turn off the faucet without touching the faucet. Toss the paper towel into the wastebasket without touching the wastebasket.

12. Be sure to apply hand lotion. Soap tends to be very drying to the skin.

HANDWASHING TO NEW HEIGHTS

Directions: Starting at the bottom of the list, circle the steps that were completed properly, working to the top of the ladder.

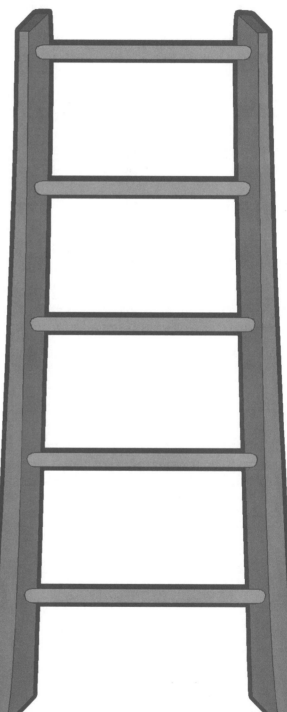

- turned off faucet without touching it

- dried hands with a clean towel

- dropped soap into soapdish

- used friction

- washed for one to two minutes, started at the fingertips and worked toward the forearms

- gave special care to thumbs, sides of fingers, knuckles, sides of the hands, and under the fingernails

- used adequate soap/worked up a good lather

- wet hands and wrists under running water

- held the bar of soap during washing

- rinsed the bar of soap before using it

- turned on warm, running water

HANDWASHING FOR HEALTHY HANDS

Treasure Chest

"Handwashing For
Healthy Hands"

"How To Handwash"

Soap

Towel

Paper towel

Access to water

Orange stick or nail file

Hand lotion

PREPARATION

1. Copy "Handwashing For Healthy Hands."
2. Copy and review "How To Handwash."
3. Be sure the patient has access to clean water, soap, and clean towel.

IMPLEMENTATION

1. Explain proper handwashing technique to the patient. Refer to "How To Handwash."
2. Reinforce the importance of proper handwashing by reviewing "Handwashing For Healthy Hands."
3. Have the patient demonstrate proper handwashing *after* you demonstrate the proper technique.
4. Leave "Handwashing For Healthy Hands" with the patient.

By: Billie Phillips, MSN, RN

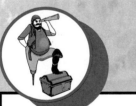

Educator Insights

"Handwashing For
Healthy Hands" and "How
To Handwash" are
excellent teaching tools
for patients with limited
reading and writing skills.

HANDWASHING FOR HEALTHY HANDS

THIS IS A GERM.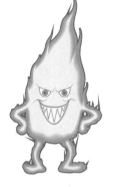

GERMS CANNNOT BE SEEN BY THE 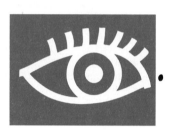.

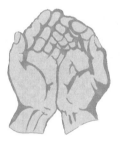 + 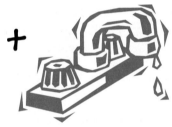 IS THE MOST

IMPORTANT THING YOU CAN DO TO PREVENT

THE SPREAD OF 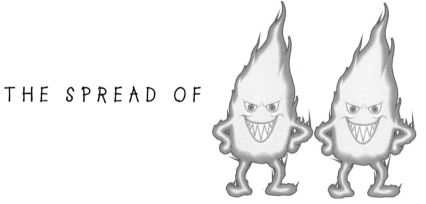 WHICH CAUSE

ILLNESS AND DISEASE.

114

HOW TO HANDWASH

USE [soap] AND WARM [water].

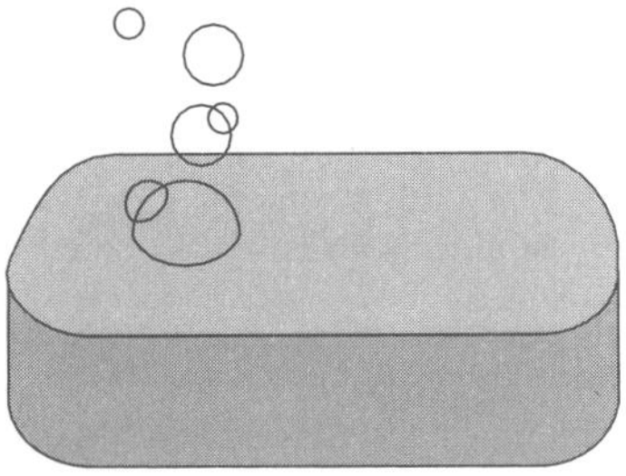

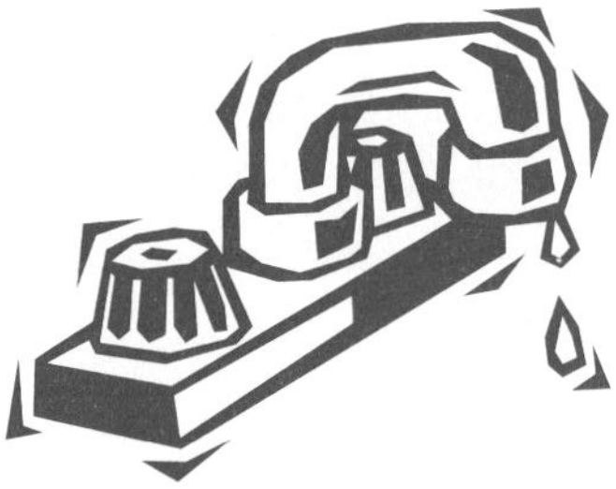

LATHER AND RUB [hands] TO A COUNT

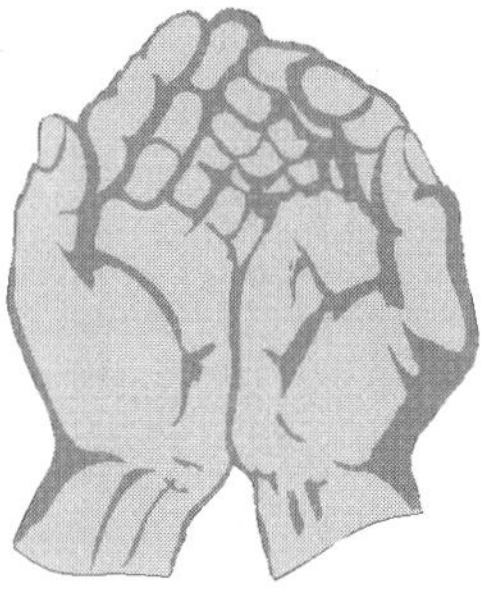

OF **"10".** BE SURE TO CLEAN

INSIDE YOUR [hand] AND

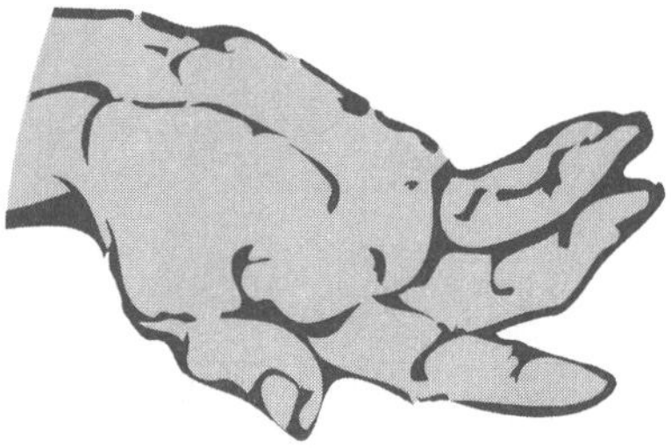

UNDER YOUR NAILS. RINSE AND DRY WITH

A CLEAN [towel].

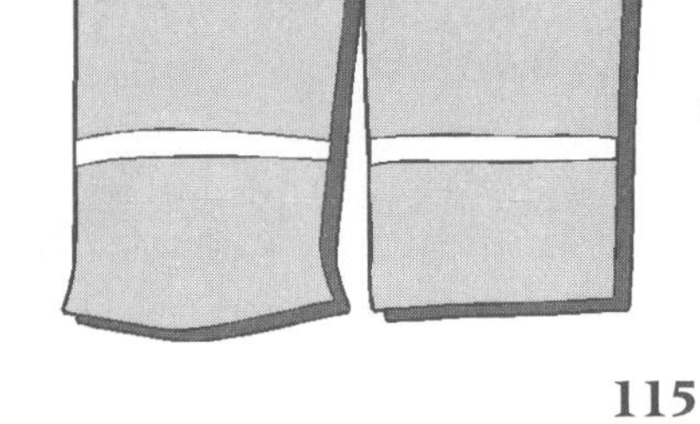

115

REMEMBER:

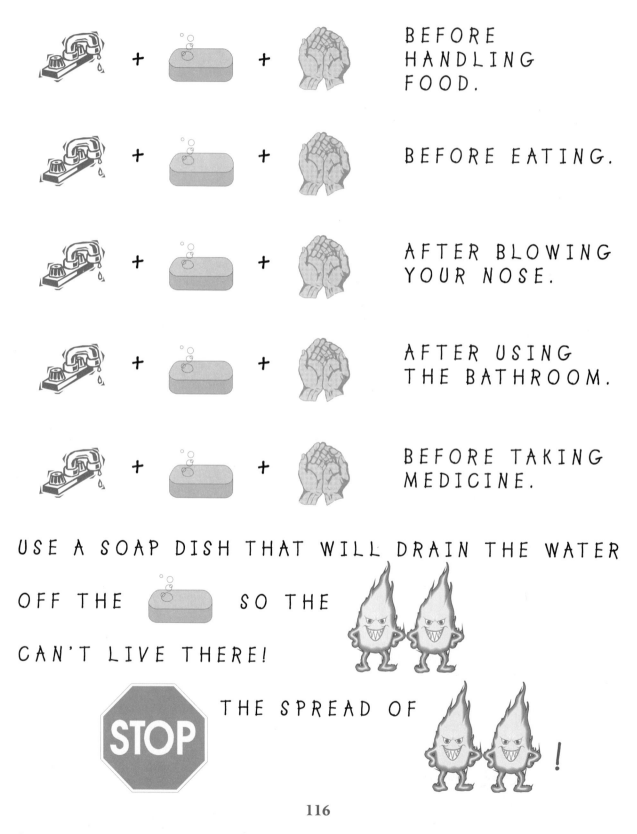

BEFORE HANDLING FOOD.

BEFORE EATING.

AFTER BLOWING YOUR NOSE.

AFTER USING THE BATHROOM.

BEFORE TAKING MEDICINE.

USE A SOAP DISH THAT WILL DRAIN THE WATER OFF THE   SO THE   CAN'T LIVE THERE!

STOP   THE SPREAD OF   !

116

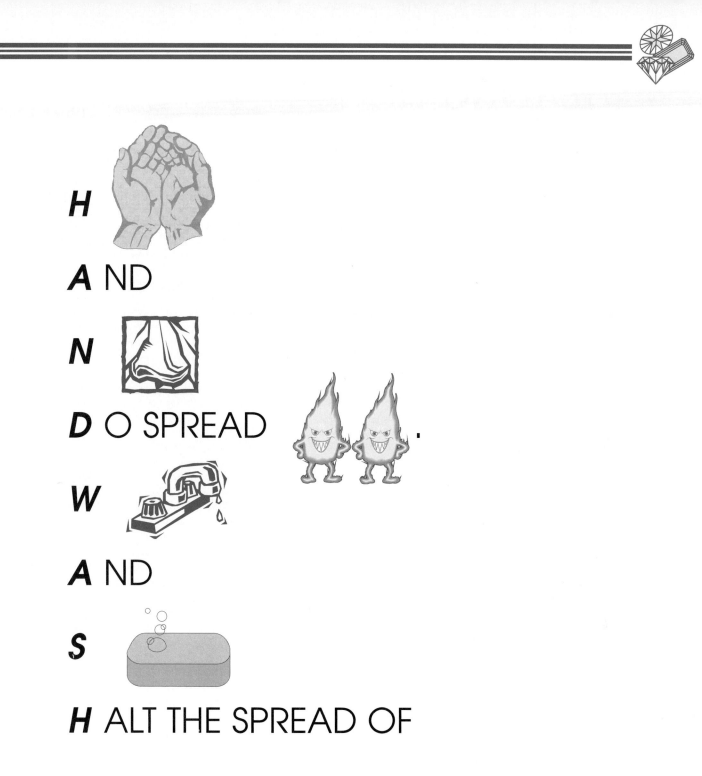

H

A ND

N

D O SPREAD .

W

A ND

S

H ALT THE SPREAD OF

I CKY

N ASTY

G 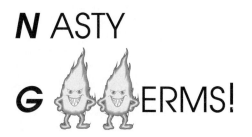 ERMS!

117

HEALING UP

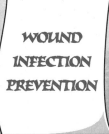

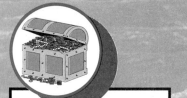

Treasure Chest

"Healing Up"

"Wound Infection Prevention" facts

"Wound Infection Warning Signs"

PREPARATION

1. Copy and review "Healing Up."
2. Copy and review "Wound Infection Prevention" facts.
3. Copy and review "Wound Infection Warning Signs."

IMPLEMENTATION

1. Discuss "Healing Up" and "Wound Infection Prevention" facts with the patient and/or caregiver.
2. Ask the patient and/or caregiver to identify wound site(s).
3. Discuss and review "Wound Infection Warning Signs" with the patient and/or caregiver.
4. Review with the patient and/or caregiver the protocol for notifying the patient's doctor or nurse.
5. Leave "Healing Up" with the patient.

By: Mary Ann Canterberry, RN, MSN

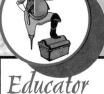

Educator Insights

If the wound is a fresh, post-op wound, instruct the patient and/or caregiver that some pain and tenderness at the wound site is normal.

HEALING UP

Preventing Wound Infection

A "wound" is considered any area on your body where your skin has been cut, torn, or broken in some way. This may be an incision site where you had surgery. It may be the open area around your tracheostomy or breathing tube. It may be the site where a feeding tube goes into your stomach. It could be a bedsore.

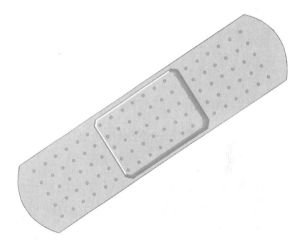

Wherever the site of the wound, there must be an all out effort to keep the wound free from infection. A wound infection is a wound that has organisms or tiny life forms, usually bacteria, growing in it.

My wound is _____

It is located on _____

The wound treatment prescribed by my doctor is:

_____

_____

_____

119

Wound Infection Prevention

1. In persons with a wound, bacterial wound contamination or infection is a common occurrence.

2. If you have a wound, you should watch the wound for signs of possible infection.

3. For your wound to become infected, you must come in contact with an infecting agent or germ. This "infecting" agent is usually a bacteria.

4. Because bacteria live all around us, it is possible for anyone's wound to become infected.

5. Bacteria are usually transferred from person to person by air currents. This can happen when we cough, sneeze, or shake dirty bed linens.

6. Cover your mouth and nose with a tissue when you cough, sneeze, or blow your nose.

7. Have others with whom you come in contact cover their mouth and nose when they cough, sneeze, or blow their nose.

8. When changing your bed, don't shake the "dirty" bed linens. This is just another way to spread germs.

9. Bacteria can also be carried from place to place by dirty hands.

10. Wash your hands before and after you touch your wound or the skin around it. Handwashing will help decrease your risk for wound infection.

11. Tell those who touch your wound or the skin around it to wash their hands before and after they touch the wound.

12. Cleanse and dress the wound exactly as the doctor orders.

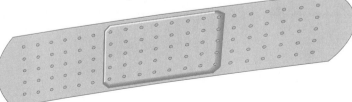

120

WOUND INFECTION

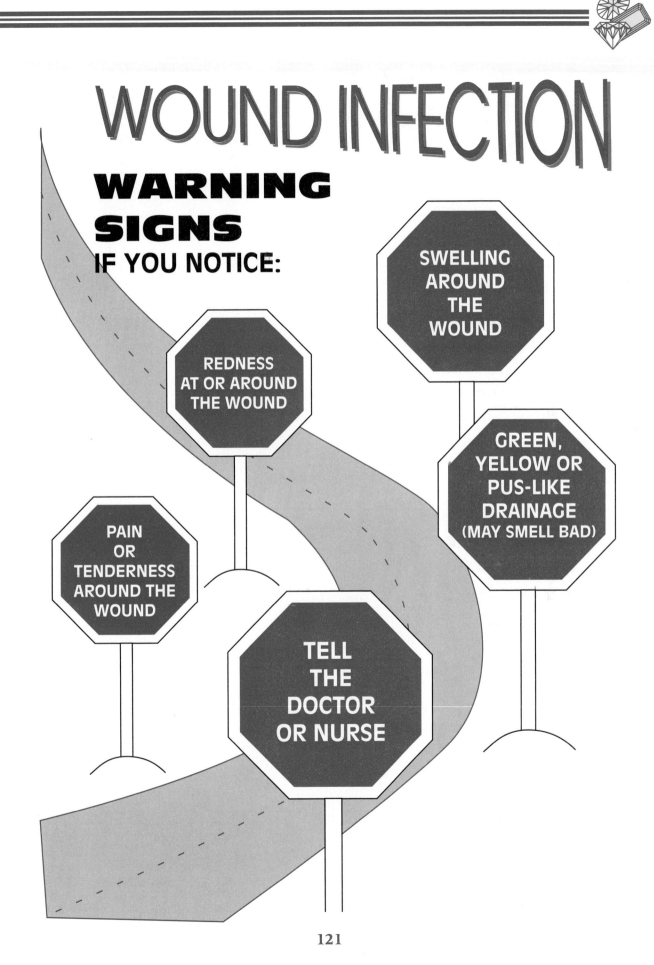

WARNING SIGNS

IF YOU NOTICE:

SWELLING AROUND THE WOUND

REDNESS AT OR AROUND THE WOUND

GREEN, YELLOW OR PUS-LIKE DRAINAGE (MAY SMELL BAD)

PAIN OR TENDERNESS AROUND THE WOUND

TELL THE DOCTOR OR NURSE

121

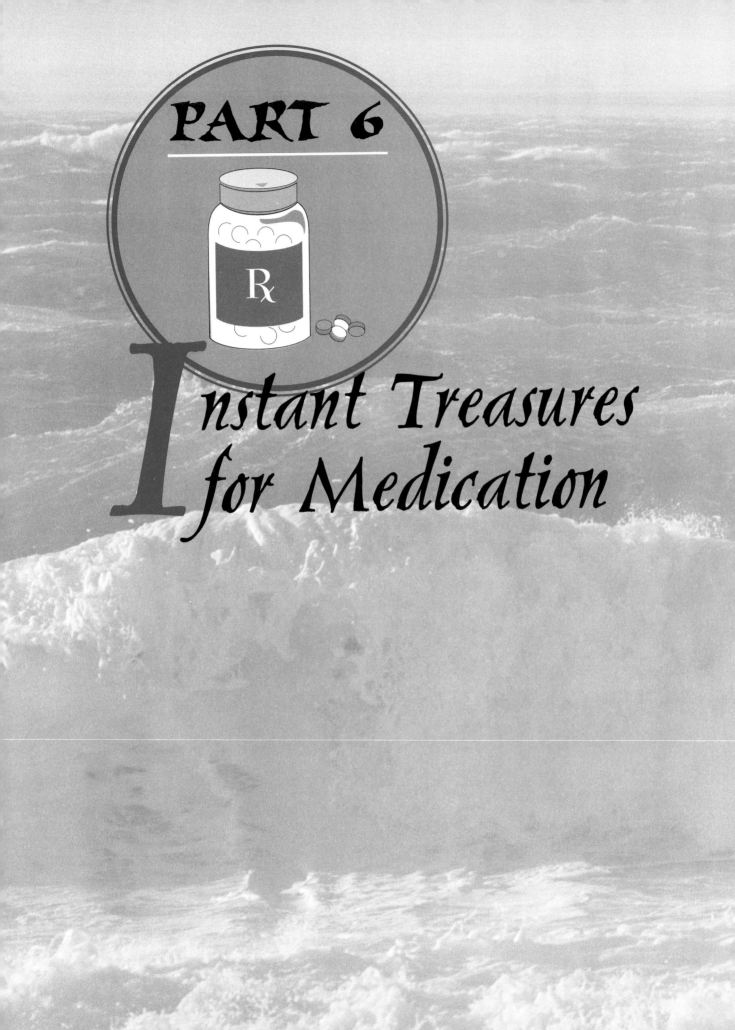

PART 6

Instant Treasures for Medication

MEDICATION MUSTS

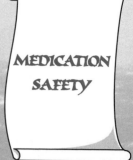

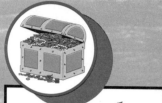

Treasure Chest

"Medication Musts: (To The Patient Teacher)"

"Medication Musts"

Medication set-up device

Empty egg carton

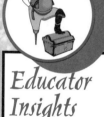

Educator Insights

Use the patient's own medications as icons as you teach.

PREPARATION

1. Review "Medication Musts: (To The Patient Teacher)."
2. Copy and review "Medication Musts."
3. Obtain a medication set-up device for demonstration purposes. (Many pharmacies have a variety of types for under five dollars.)

IMPLEMENTATION

1. Discuss "Medication Musts" with the patient.
2. Show the sample medication set-up device and tell the patient the cost and where one can be purchased.
3. If a "store-bought" device is not an option, assist the patient in making one from an egg carton.
4. If an egg carton is used, clearly label each compartment. Be sure to find a covering for the egg carton. A cake plate lid may work.
5. Assist the patient to locate a safe place for storage of medications, out of the reach of children.
6. Keep in mind that medications should not be stored in a place that is too hot or excessively moist.
7. Review "Medication Musts" with the patient.
8. Leave "Medication Musts" with the patient.

By: Gaye Ragland, RN, BSN

Medication Musts:
(To The Patient Teacher)

For many patients, taking medications each day is as much a part of their routine as eating meals at mealtime. Yet many patients take incorrect dosages, stop taking the medication if they begin to feel better, and fail to take doses at the intervals prescribed.

If medications are to be taken properly, it is essential that the patient has a system for remembering to take medications exactly as prescribed. Inform the patient and/or caregivers of the various types of medication "set-up" devices that are available. Several types are available at most local pharmacies. Empty egg cartons work well as medication containers if a "store-bought" one is not an option. If an egg carton is used, mark the pockets clearly with the names and times the medications are to be taken. Also, find a way to cover the open egg carton between times for medications so the patient can simply pick the covering up without disturbing the carton (a clear plastic dish or a cake cover may work).

Be sure to include proper storage of medications as you teach medication musts. Instruct the patient to store medications in a safe place. Remind the patient that the years of "child-proofing" the home may be many years past. Many elderly patients, however, may keep grandchildren or have visits from them. It is a must that medications be kept out of the reach of children. Low counters in the patient's bathroom are accessible to small children. Assist the patient, if necessary, to find a safe storage place for medications and away from excessive moisture or heat.

MEDICATION MUSTS

✔ Take all medication exactly as it is prescribed by your doctor.

✔ Take the medication until it is finished.

✔ Do not stop taking the prescribed medication just because you begin to feel better. Many medications have not finished doing the work until the entire prescription is taken.

✔ Do not share your medication with anyone else.

✔ Do not take extra medication thinking, "If one pill made me some better, then two pills will make me feel a lot better."

✔ Do not keep unused medication. If your medication is discontinued, discard it.

✔ If you forget to take a medication, do not double the dose the next time.

✔ If you have new symptoms after taking your medication, notify your physician or nurse immediately.

✔ Your pharmacist can answer questions about your medication. The telephone number of your pharmacy is usually printed on the pill bottle.

✔ Do not mix alcohol with medications unless you have approval from your doctor.

126

MEDICATION EDUCATION

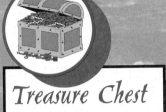

Treasure Chest

"Medication Education"

Current medication reference book

Pen or pencil with an eraser

Educator Insights

Be sure to include the generic name of the drug if it is different from the brand name.

PREPARATION

1. Copy "Medication Education."
2. Look up in a current drug reference book the drug to be taught and review information about the drug.
3. Review the patient's medication regimen for other drugs, foods, or alcohol that may interact with the medication.
4. Call the pharmacist for additional information, if needed.
5. Make sure the patient has a pen or pencil with an eraser.

IMPLEMENTATION

1. Have the medication being taught in hand.
2. Encourage the patient to hold the container. Verify for correctness as you both look at the label.
3. Complete the "Medication Education" form by filling in the blanks.
4. As you teach, be concrete and specific. Keep sentences short. Keep explanations to a minimum. Ask the patient to repeat, or read from the sheet, what you have discussed.
5. Reinforce "Medication Education" on future visits.
6. Leave "Medication Education" with the patient.

By: Gaye Ragland, RN, BSN

MEDICATION EDUCATION

Patient's name: _____.

Name of the medication: _____.

Doctor who prescribed it: _____.

Purpose of the medication: _____.

Is the medication to be taken with food, milk, or on an empty stomach? ____

_____

When is the medication to be taken? _____

_____

If the medication is ordered for times around mealtime, how long before or after meals is it to be taken? (Specify if it is to be taken with meals.) _____

_____

Are there special instructions about the storage of this medication? _____

_____

Will this medication be taken for just a short period or will this prescription need to be refilled until my doctor or nurse tells me otherwise? _____

_____

Probable side effects: _____

_____

Possible side effects: _____

_____

Who to report side effects to: _____ phone # _____

Warnings about food, alcohol and other drugs to be avoided: _____

_____

DON'T MONKEY AROUND WITH YOUR MEDICATION

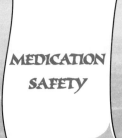

MEDICATION SAFETY

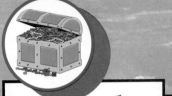

Treasure Chest

"Don't Monkey Around With Your Medication" exercise

"Don't Monkey Around With Your Medication" answer key

Pen or pencil with an eraser

PREPARATION

1. Copy "Don't Monkey Around With Your Medication" exercise.
2. Copy "Don't Monkey Around With Your Medication" answer key.
3. Make sure the patient has a pen or pencil with an eraser.

IMPLEMENTATION

1. Have the patient complete "Don't Monkey Around With Your Medication" exercise.
2. Point out the word bank at the bottom of the exercise. Words can only be used once.
3. Use the answer key to check the patient's work.
4. Correct and explain any missed answers.
5. Leave "Don't Monkey Around With Your Medication" with the patient.

By: Gaye Ragland, RN, BSN

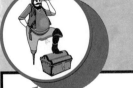

Educator Insights

To prevent the patient from acting on incorrect information **do not** leave this treasure with the patient until it is completed and checked for accuracy. This exercise is designed to be completed **with** the patient.

DON'T MONKEY AROUND WITH YOUR MEDICATION

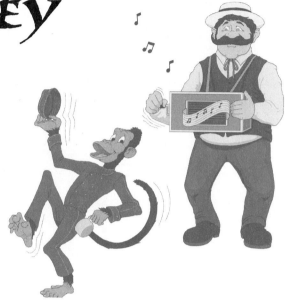

Directions: Complete the following warnings by filling in the blanks. Choose the words from the word bank at the bottom of the next page.

1. Be sure to take the RIGHT _____.

2. Be sure to take your medication at the RIGHT _____.

3. Be sure to take your medication for the RIGHT number of _____.
   Take all that is prescribed for you for the length of time your doctor ordered.

4. Be sure to take your medication with _____ or _____,
   if that is how the doctor ordered it.

5. Be sure to keep your medication out of the reach of _____.

6. Be sure your medication is stored in a place where it will not get too much _____ or get too _____.

7. If you forget to take your medication, do not _____ the dose the next time.

8. Some medications are ordered to be taken around _____. If so, take your medication according to the doctor's orders.

9. Do not stop taking your medication just because you feel _____. You should take it all, unless otherwise ordered.

10. If you develop new symptoms after taking your medication, notify the _____ or _____.

11. If your medication is discontinued, _____ it.

12. Do not give your prescription medication to other _____.

13. If you have questions about your medication, you may call your _____.

14. Ask your _____ about any food, other medication, or alcohol that should not be mixed with your medication.

WORD BANK			
MEDICATION	DOUBLE	MEALTIME	CHILDREN
DOCTOR	NURSE	FOOD OR MILK	BETTER
HOT	DISCARD	PHARMACIST	PHARMACIST
DAYS	TIME	PEOPLE	MOISTURE

DON'T MONKEY AROUND WITH YOUR MEDICATION

ANSWER KEY:

1. Be sure to take the RIGHT _____ **MEDICATION** _____ .

2. Be sure to take your medication at the RIGHT _____ **TIME** _____ .

3. Be sure to take your medication for the RIGHT number of __**DAYS**__ . Take all that is prescribed for you for the length of time your doctor ordered.

4. Be sure to take your medication with ___**FOOD**___ or _____**MILK**_____ , if that is how the doctor ordered it.

5. Be sure to keep your medication out of the reach of ___**CHILDREN**___ .

6. Be sure your medication is stored in a place where it will not get too much _____**MOISTURE**_____ or get too _____**HOT**_____ .

7. If you forget to take your medication, do not _____ **DOUBLE** _____ the dose the next time.

132

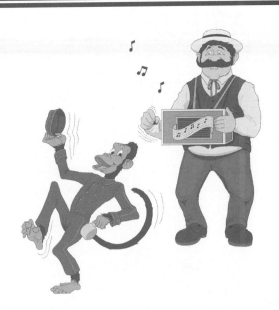

8. Some medications are ordered to be taken around __MEALTIME__. If so, take your medication according to the doctor's orders.

9. Do not stop taking medication just because you feel __BETTER__. You should take it all, unless otherwise ordered.

10. If you develop new symptoms after taking your medication, notify the _____NURSE_____ or _____DOCTOR_____.

11. If your medication is discontinued, _____DISCARD_____ it.

12. Do not give your prescription medication to other __PEOPLE__.

13. If you have questions about your medication, you may call your _____PHARMACIST_____.

14. Ask your _____PHARMACIST_____ about any food, other medication, or alcohol that should not be mixed with your medication.

MEDICATION MEMO

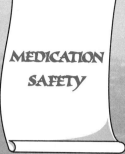

MEDICATION SAFETY

PREPARATION

1. Copy "Medication Memo."
2. Depending on the number of medications the patient is taking, more than one copy of the "Medication Memo" may be needed.
3. If a hot glue gun is used, plug it in for several minutes before it is needed to allow the glue to warm and soften (optional).
4. Make sure caregiver has pen or pencil with an eraser.

IMPLEMENTATION

1. Complete "Medication Memo" by filling in the date the list is completed, the roster of medications, your signature and title and the name of the patient's physician and physician's telephone number.
2. OPTIONAL ACTIVITY: Beside the name of each medication listed on the "Medication Memo," glue a sample of the corresponding pill. Additional information, such as, the generic name, brand name, dosage, time, and reason for taking the medication may be included on the medication memo. **Be sure to obtain permission for using the patient's pills before starting this activity. If it is necessary to glue pills beside the corresponding name of the medication, the memo must be kept out of the reach of children at all times.**
3. Some patients prefer to keep this list in their purse. Other patients prefer to keep this list in the kitchen or near their meds.
4. If the patient chooses to post the list, remind the patient that the list can be viewed by anyone coming into that area of the home.
5. Keep the list updated as medications change.
6. When completed, leave the medication list with the patient.

By: Gaye Ragland, RN, BSN

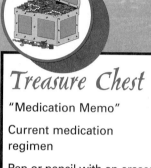

Treasure Chest

"Medication Memo"

Current medication regimen

Pen or pencil with an eraser

Hot glue gun (optional)

Hot glue sticks (optional)

Educator Insights

With the patient's approval, the "Medication Memo" left in a conspicuous place (i.e., refrigerator) could be of great assistance to emergency medical services.

Medication Memo

YOUR CURRENT MEDICATIONS AS OF _____ .

TODAY'S DATE

1. _____
2. _____
3. _____
4. _____
5. _____
6. _____
7. _____
8. _____
9. _____
10. _____
11. _____
12. _____

Pharmacy Name: _____

Pharmacy Number: _____

_____

Signature and Title

_____

Physician's Name

_____

Physician's Number

135

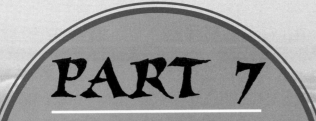

PART 7

Instant Treasures for Personal Care

POTS AND PANS

PREPARATION

1. Copy and review "Pots and Pans."
2. Obtain a bottle of nail polish and remover.
3. Make sure the caregiver has a pen or pencil with an eraser.

IMPLEMENTATION

1. Discuss "Pots and Pans" with the patient and/or caregiver.
2. Help find something the patient can use as a call bell. If the patient or caregiver does not have a bell, a small pan and spoon can be banged together to make noise when the patient is finished and needing help.
3. Demonstrate the front of bedpan and how to roll the patient who cannot help on to the bedpan. Talk about friction, the damage it can cause to the skin, and how to prevent it.
4. Demonstrate giving the bedpan using good body mechanics. Point out to the caregiver good body mechanic techniques as you use them, then have the caregiver demonstrate them.
5. Leave "Pots and Pans" in the home with the caregiver.

By: Gaye Ragland, RN, BSN

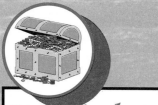

Treasure Chest

"Pots and Pans (and urinals, too)"

Nail polish and nail polish remover

Pen or pencil with an eraser

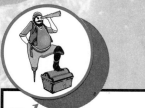

Educator Insights

Use nail polish and remover as a teaching icon to demonstrate friction. After polishing one fingernail, wait several minutes for it to dry. Then using a small amount of remover, demonstrate the "rubbing away" of a thin layer by rubbing the polish off the fingernail.

Pots and Pans

(and Urinals, Too)

For the patient who is unable to get up and down to the bathroom, or for the patient who sometimes has problems getting all the way to the bathroom, the bedpan, commode chair, and urinal may become required equipment. The bedpan is the pan into which a patient urinates or has a bowel movement. The commode chair is a portable toilet. It is easily moved from room to room, but usually kept at the patient's bedside. The urinal is the container into which the patient urinates.

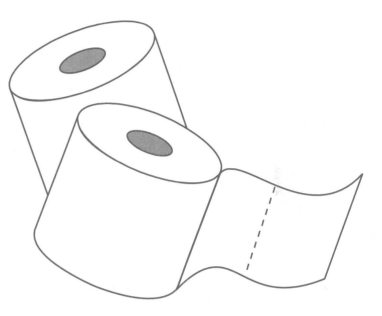

Listed below are practical tips for using pots (commode chair), pans (bedpans, that is), and urinals.

• Put the commode chair close to the patient so he/she does not have far to walk.

• Be sure the patient has privacy. Even at home all patients need bathroom privacy. If the commode chair is in the patient's bedroom, close the doors and blinds to ensure privacy. Privacy is also necessary for the patient who uses the bedpan or urinal while in the bed.

• Never leave the patient alone with no way to call you. Either remain within earshot, just outside the door, or give the patient a bell to ring.

• Put tissue in the bedpan or commode bucket before the patient uses it. The tissue will keep stool from sticking to the bottom of the pan or commode chair bucket and make clean-up at the time of emptying much easier.

• When positioning the bedpan, remember the narrow side goes in the front.

139

- Before putting the patient on the bedpan, place a towel or linen saver on the sheet under the patient's hips. Sometimes when bedpans are full, a little of the contents will spill out. If this happens you must change the wet linen immediately.

- If possible, raise the head of the bed so that the patient is in a sitting position. In the home, you may prop the patient with pillows to a sitting position, if possible.

- Sprinkle a small amount of powder on the rim of the bedpan before sliding it under the patient. This keeps the patient from sticking to the pan and lessens friction. This is easier on the patient's skin. Friction can cause damage to the skin.

- Have the patient turn on his side or lift his hips. Slide the pan under the patient with the wide end toward the back. Check to be sure the pan is centered under the patient. Help the patient into a sitting position, if possible. Check to be sure the pan is in the right position once under the patient.

- When the patient is finished, put on gloves. Clean the patient with tissue, if necessary.

- Raise the side rails before leaving the room. CAUTION: Because the caregiver is focusing on emptying the waste at this time, it is easy to forget to raise the rails. REMEMBER: Raise the rails.

- Cover the bucket from the commode chair, the bedpan, or the urinal as soon as you take it from the patient. Carry it covered to the toilet. Remove the urine and bowel movement (stool) from the room immediately.

- Help the patient wash his/her hands. Wash your hands.

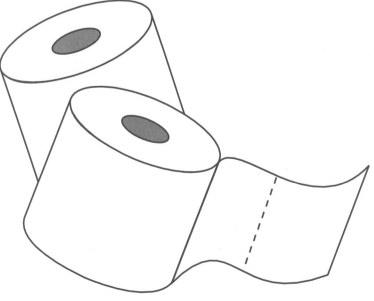

POTS AND PANS CROSSWORD PUZZLE

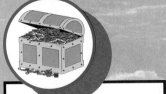

Treasure Chest

"Pots and Pans" crossword puzzle

"Pots and Pans" crossword puzzle answer key

Pen or pencil with an eraser

Small reward (optional)

PREPARATION

1. Copy "Pots and Pans" crossword puzzle.
2. Copy "Pots and Pans" crossword puzzle answer key.
3. Obtain a small reward.
4. Make sure the caregiver has a pen or pencil with an eraser.

IMPLEMENTATION

1. Ask the patient and/or caregiver to complete the "Pots and Pans" crossword puzzle.
2. Explain that the answers to the questions may be found in the fact sheet, "Pots and Pans."
3. Check the answers to the puzzle with the patient or caregiver when finished or leave the answer sheet (folded together with the answers out of view). The patient and/or caregiver may check the answers whenever the crossword puzzle is completed.
4. Leave "Pots and Pans" crossword puzzle and answer key with the caregiver.

By: Gaye Ragland, RN, BSN

Educator Insights

A roll of toilet tissue is a great reward and good for a hearty laugh!

POTS and PANS (AND URINALS, TOO!)
Crossword Puzzle

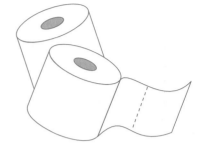

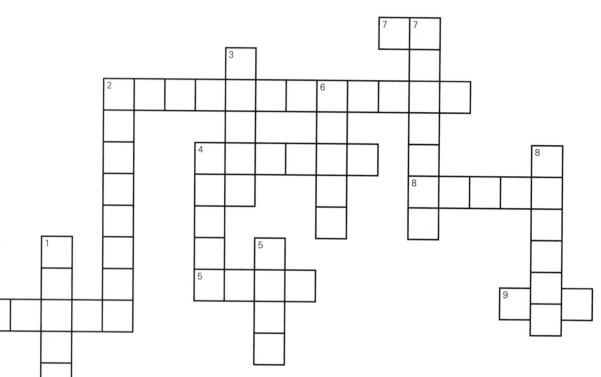

ACROSS

2. A portable commode.
3. This often happens when you remove the bedpan.
4. _____ the bedpan from the room as quickly as possible.
5. Friction from the bedpan can damage the patient's _____.
7. Before leaving the patient's bed, remember to pull the bedrail _____.
8. _____ the blinds or door for privacy.
9. Which gender most often uses the urinal?

DOWN

1. Container into which the (usually male) patient urinates.
2. What to leave with the patient if you leave the room.
3. _____ the patient's body to ensure privacy.
4. Raise the _____.
5. On most bedpans, the back side is low, the front side is _____.
6. _____ the bedpan, urinal, or bucket from the commode chair before you carry it out of the room.
7. Always try to maintain the patient's _____.
8. A device the patient may use to urinate in while in bed.

142

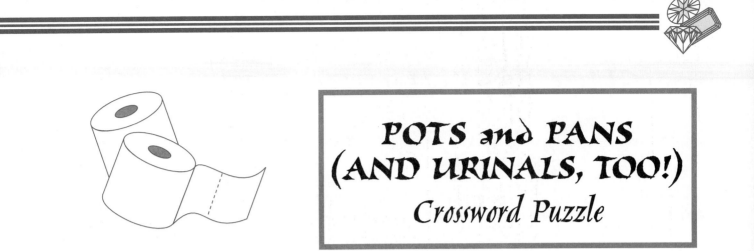

POTS and PANS (AND URINALS, TOO!)
Crossword Puzzle

ANSWER KEY:

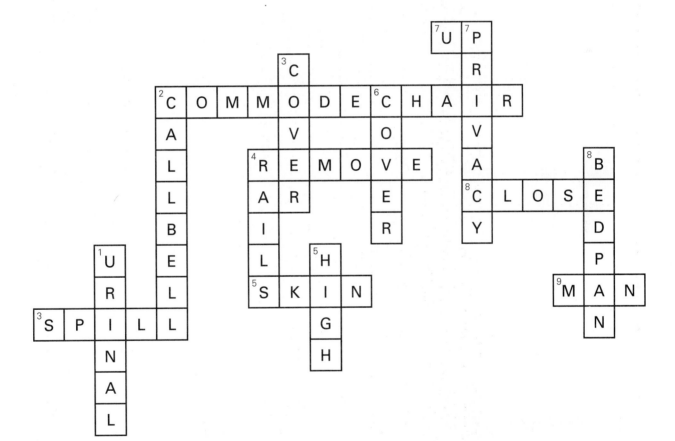

10 STEPS TO SUCCESSFUL BLADDER TRAINING

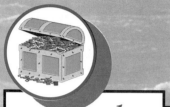

PREPARATION

1. Copy and review "Ten Steps to Successful Bladder Training."
2. Copy "Here We Go Kegeling Along."

Treasure Chest

"Ten Steps to Successful Bladder Training"

"Here We Go Kegeling Along"

IMPLEMENTATION

1. Discuss "Ten Steps to Successful Bladder Training" with the patient and caregiver.
2. Write specifics of the program in the designated area on page 2 of the "Ten Steps" fact sheet.
3. Teach Kegel exercises for better bladder control.
4. Offer encouragement and praise for the patient's acceptance of the challenge.
5. Leave "10 Steps to Successful Bladder Training" with the caregiver.
6. Leave "Here We Go Kegeling Along" with the patient/caregiver.

By: Susan Lofton, MSN, RN

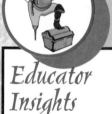

Educator Insights

Kegel exercises can be reviewed in most medical-surgical textbooks. Get ready to share a laugh as you and the patient sing the song.

10 Steps to SUCCESSFUL Bladder Training

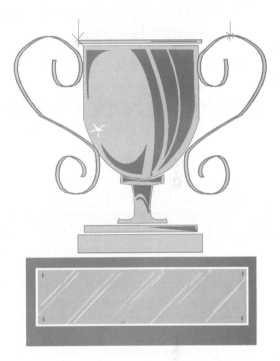

1. Develop **PATIENCE** . . . this is the essential ingredient on everyone's part. Sit down and develop a game plan before starting the actual bladder training.

2. Make sure your training program includes **drinking enough fluids** . . . withholding fluids is the worst possible approach to bladder training!

3. Carefully develop specific **voiding or urinating schedules.** Take your loved one to the toilet at least every two hours. Provide plenty of privacy and time for your patient to void.

4. **Never scold or fuss** your patient about accidents. "No use crying over spilt urine!"

5. During the training, **pad the bed or clothing** to protect against wetness. Try to **avoid diapering,** as this may falsely give "permission" to be incontinent or wet the diaper.

6. **Offer your patient fluids** every two hours throughout the day. This will help stimulate the reflex needed to control the bladder.

7. You may **limit fluids during the later evening hours** to allow longer sleep periods at night.

8. Have your patient **avoid caffeine products.** Caffeine contributes to bladder irritability.

9. **Kegel** exercises are a great way to improve bladder tone. Ask your patient to "hold" their urine mid-stream by contracting the bladder muscles tightly for a count of three. Contract. Count to three. Release the urine flow. This may be increased to the count of ten. Complete these exercises at least four times each day when urinating.

10. **Praise and encourage your patient frequently. Never criticize your patient's failures.**

SPECIAL BLADDER TRAINING INSTRUCTIONS:

_____

_____

_____

_____

_____

_____

_____

_____

"HERE WE . . . GO KEGELING . . . ALONG"

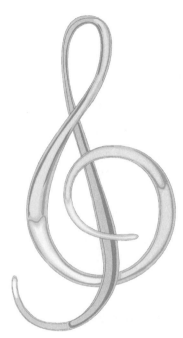

Sing to the tune of:
"The Caissons Go Rolling Along"

. . . Over Hill, Over Dale
. . . we will leave no urine trail . . .
. . . cause we Kegel, we Kegel along . . .

. . . Urine flows, Urine stops . . .
. . . As we count without a clock . . .
. . . As we Kegel, we Kegel along . . .

. . . Hi . . . Hi . . . He . . .
. . . we count from one to three . . .
. . . holding those muscles TIGHT and STRONG . . .

. . . We will never give in . . .
. . . holding tight from one to ten . . .
. . . as we Kegel, we Kegel along!

147

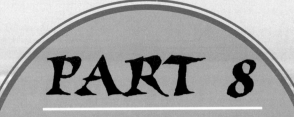

PART 8

FIRE

Instant Treasures for Patient Safety

SAFETY IS GOLDEN

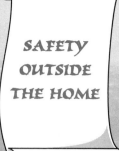

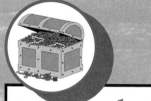

Treasure Chest

"Golden Safety Tips"

"Safety Checklist"

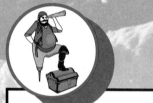

Educator Insights

Over 4,000 senior citizens will be criminally victimized in their homes, 425 will be raped, and 11 will be attacked in their driveway each day.

Source: Mizell, L. R., 1994.

PREPARATION

1. Review and copy "Golden Safety Tips."
2. Copy "Safety Checklist."

IMPLEMENTATION

1. Discuss with the patient the need for safety awareness when the patient leaves the home.
2. Use the "Golden Safety Tips" sheet to teach the patient about basic safety actions.
3. Leave the "Golden Safety Tips" sheet with the patient and place the "Safety Checklist" sheet near the home entrance for the patient and caregiver to check as a reminder before they leave home.

*By: Paul A. Davey, M.S., LPC and
Debrynda B. Davey, Ed.D., RN*

Golden Safety Tips

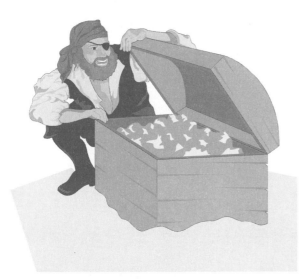

✓ **Wear seatbelts.**

✓ **Lock car doors.**

✓ **Keep control of keys.**

✓ **Carry your purse in front, close to your body.**

✓ **Stay alert. Be prepared.**

✓ **Lock your home when outside.**

✓ **Don't *look* like a victim.**

✓ **Don't give information to strangers.**

✓ **Trust your instincts.**

✓ **Don't put your name and address on keys.**

✓ **Don't go outside alone.**

✓ **Don't count or flash your money in public.**

✓ **Know your neighbors.**

✓ **Wear non-skid shoes.**

✓ **Dial 911 for help.**

Safety Checklist

☐ **Remember . . . Safety First!**

☐ **Don't take chances.**

☐ **Be alert and prepared.**

☐ **Trust your instincts.**

☐ **Don't go out alone.**

☐ **Wear non-skid shoes.**

☐ **Carry purse in front of body.**

☐ **Lock your home.**

☐ **Wear your seatbelt.**

☐ **Lock your car doors.**

☐ **Don't talk to strangers!**

IT TAKES THREE THINGS TO START A FIRE

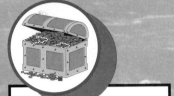

FIRE SAFETY

Treasure Chest

"It Takes Three Things To Start A Fire"

"Fuel That Fire"

"Fuel That Fire" answer sheet

Orange highlighter

Pen or pencil with an eraser

Educator Insights

Have the patient verbalize a fire evacuation plan from each room of the home.

PREPARATION

1. Copy and review "It Takes Three Things To Start A Fire."
2. Copy "Fuel That Fire."
3. Copy "Fuel That Fire" answer sheet.
4. Make sure with a pen or pencil with an eraser.

IMPLEMENTATION

1. Use "It Takes Three Things to Start a Fire" to explain the fire triangle to the patient.
2. Talk about each of the three elements of the fire triangle and give examples of each.
3. Ask the patient to complete the word search puzzle.
4. Explain that the hidden words are words associated with things that will burn.
5. Help the patient conclude that almost all things in the home may be fuel, that oxygen is ever present and that carelessness with a match or spark can create a devastating, accidental fire.
6. Check the patient's answers.
7. Leave "It Takes Three Things To Start A Fire" with the patient.

By: Gaye Ragland, RN, BSN

IT TAKES THREE THINGS TO START A FIRE.

THE FIRE TRIANGLE IS SHOWN BELOW:

OXYGEN

THE AIR WE BREATHE

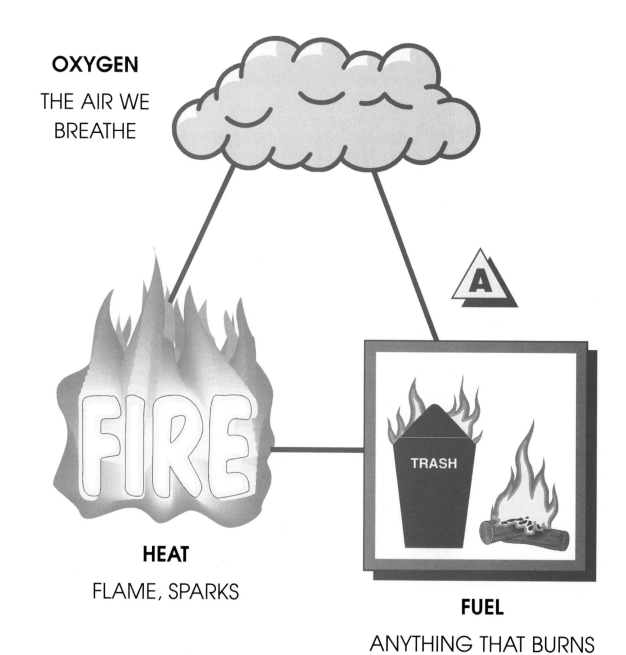

HEAT

FLAME, SPARKS

TRASH

FUEL

ANYTHING THAT BURNS

154

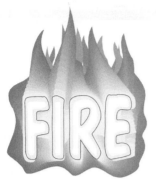

FUEL THAT FIRE
Word Search

Directions: Using an orange marker, highlight each of the hidden words that would **"FUEL THAT FIRE."**

Remember: The words can be forward, backward, up and down, and diagonal.

T	D	O	O	W	E	R	I	F	J	P	H	C
A	S	X	G	A	R	B	A	G	E	A	R	A
B	A	T	H	R	O	B	E	N	H	N	A	N
L	E	A	V	E	S	P	M	D	H	T	E	D
E	M	A	G	A	Z	I	N	E	S	S	W	L
E	B	N	W	O	G	T	H	G	I	N	R	E
O	L	D	R	A	G	S	P	E	C	E	E	S
N	E	W	S	P	A	P	E	R	Y	N	D	S
H	S	S	A	R	G	A	S	O	L	I	N	E
P	G	H	R	I	A	H	C	N	H	L	U	O
M	O	N	I	S	J	A	O	P	H	D	L	H
A	W	V	C	R	G	I	A	M	D	E	M	S
L	N	C	O	V	T	R	T	G	Z	B	N	L

WORDS:

Tables	Bed Linen	Shirt	Magazines	Pants
Newspaper	Nightgown	Bathrobe	Candles	Firewood
Underwear	Gasoline	Shoes	Garbage	Old Rags
Chair	Grass	Coat	Leaves	
Lamp	Bed	Hair	Gown	

155

FUEL THAT FIRE
Word Search

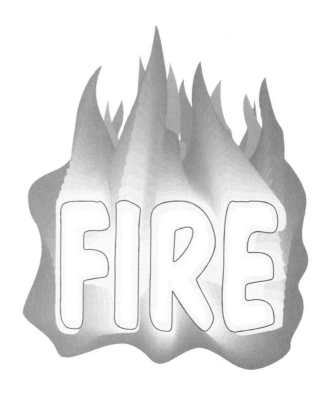

ANSWER KEY:

T	D	O	O	W	E	R	I	F	J	P	H	C
A	S	X	G	A	R	B	A	G	E	A	R	A
B	A	T	H	R	O	B	E	N	H	N	A	N
L	E	A	V	E	S	P	M	D	H	T	E	D
E	M	A	G	A	Z	I	N	E	S	S	W	L
E	B	N	W	O	G	T	H	G	I	N	R	E
O	L	D	R	A	G	S	P	E	C	E	E	S
N	E	W	S	P	A	P	E	R	Y	N	D	S
H	S	S	A	R	G	A	S	O	L	I	N	E
P	G	H	R	I	A	H	C	N	H	L	U	O
M	O	N	I	S	J	A	O	P	H	D	L	H
A	W	V	C	R	G	I	A	M	D	E	M	S
L	N	C	O	V	T	R	T	G	Z	B	N	L

156

BREATHING EASY

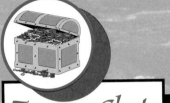

Treasure Chest

"Breathing Easy"

"A Visit from Cousin Verne"

Educator Insights

Review adjusting the flowmeter with the patient. If the biprongs are too long for your patient's comfort, clip with nail clippers as needed for a comfortable fit.

PREPARATION

1. Copy and review "Breathing Easy."
2. Copy and review "A Visit From Cousin Verne."

IMPLEMENTATION

1. Review "Breathing Easy" with the patient.
2. Read "A Visit From Cousin Verne." Have the patient give the answers to the "What Do You Say When" questions.
3. Leave "Breathing Easy" with the patient.

By: Laverne Grant

Breathing Easy

Guidelines for the Use of Oxygen in the Home

Your doctor has ordered oxygen for your use at home. Listed below are some very important guidelines that you and your family need to know.

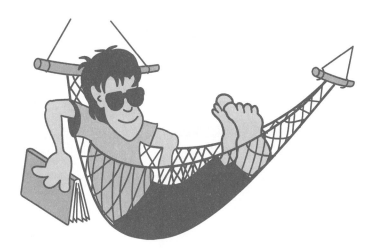

1. Do Not use oxygen near an open flame/fire.

2. Do Not smoke.

3. Do Not allow visitors to smoke.

4. Place a "NO SMOKING" sign on the door of the home and on the door of the room in which the oxygen is being used.

5. Set the flow rate at the amount your doctor prescribed. Keep the tubing free from kinks.

6. If your nose becomes dry, use a water-based lubricant (like K-Y® jelly) to soothe the irritated skin. Do **NOT** use Vaseline® or any type of oil.

7. Turn off any electrical equipment *before* it is unplugged to prevent sparks.

8. Remove any wool blankets or synthetic fabrics like nylon that could create static and cause a spark. Wear cotton clothing or pajamas.

9. Remove electrical equipment from your room (like electric razors and heating pads).

10. Remove from your room any types of substances that ignite easily. This includes oils, nail polish remover, alcohol, and any types of grease or greasy cosmetics.

11. CALL YOUR DOCTOR IF:
    - You are more restless than usual
    - You feel confused or more drowsy than usual
    - You have a lot of trouble concentrating
    - Your breathing becomes irregular
    - Your earlobes, lips, or nailbeds look blue

12. Do Not assume that more oxygen will help you breathe better.

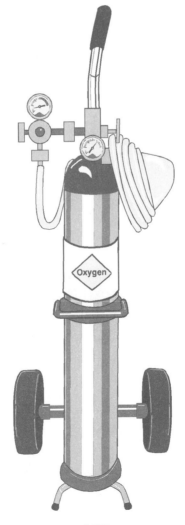

159

A VISIT FROM "COUSIN VERNE"

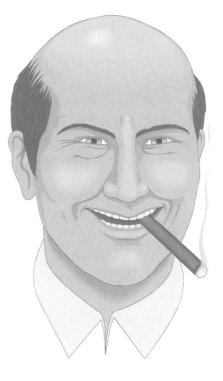

Tap . . . Tap . . . Tap at the door.
Guess who it is?
Who else but "Cousin Verne!"
Uh-oh. Cousin Verne's got his suitcase.
That means he's stayin' for a while.

DIRECTIONS: How would you respond to Cousin Verne?

WHAT DO YOU SAY WHEN:

Cousin Verne says, "You look kind of blue. Take some more oxygen. It'll do you good!"

WHAT DO YOU SAY WHEN:

Cousin Verne says, "Since we can't smoke cigarettes with the oxygen flowing, I'll just light up my cigar. That oughta be safe enough!"

WHAT DO YOU SAY WHEN:

Cousin Verne says, "We can bring your tank in here and get you good and warm, if you will let me build a fire in the fireplace, that is."

WHAT DO YOU SAY WHEN:

Cousin Verne says, "You look awfully short of breath. Let's turn that thing up a little higher."

WHAT DO YOU SAY WHEN:

Cousin Verne says, "Reach over there and snatch that TV cord out of the socket. Then plug in this electric razor and I'll give you a shave."

WHAT DO YOU SAY WHEN:

Cousin Verne says, "Your nose and lips look parched. Let me rub 'em with some vaseline. It'll do 'em good."

WHAT DO YOU SAY WHEN:

Cousin Verne says, "You need some wool pajamas. That's what you need to keep yourself warm."

WHAT DO YOU SAY WHEN:

Cousin Verne says, "Oh, don't bother to put "NO SMOKING" signs on the front door. I'll just try to remember to tell everybody."

WHAT DO YOU SAY WHEN:

Cousin Verne says, "I've really enjoyed my visit. It's time for me to go!"

THE BETTER TO SEE YOU WITH

PREPARATION

1. Copy and review "The Better To See You With."
2. Copy and review "Granny, The Glasses, And The Big, Bad Wolf."
3. Copy and review, "Curls or Girl: Can You Tell The Difference?"

IMPLEMENTATION

1. Review "The Better To See You With" with the patient.
2. Ask if the patient has a special place for eyeglasses when they are not being worn.
3. Read the story, "Granny, The Glasses, And The Big, Bad Wolf." If appropriate, vary your voice tones to liven up the story.
4. Ask the questions from the page "Curls or Girl: Can You Tell the Difference?"
5. Leave "The Better To See You With" with the patient.

By: Bonnie Davis, RN, DNS
and Gaye Ragland, RN, BSN

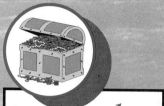

Treasure Chest

"The Better To See You With"

"Granny, The Glasses, And The Big, Bad Wolf"

"Curls or Girl: Can You Tell the Difference?"

Jumbo sunglasses (optional)

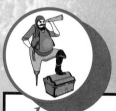

Educator Insights

Jumbo size glasses are a fun icon to wear as you teach this treasure. They are usually available at party stores for under $3.

"THE BETTER TO SEE YOU WITH"

··

Hints for the Visually Impaired

✓ **Keep your glasses clean.**

✓ **Store your glasses in the same, safe place.**

✓ **Use a magnifying glass, if needed, in addition to your glasses.**

✓ **Ask the pharmacist to use large print on medication bottles.**

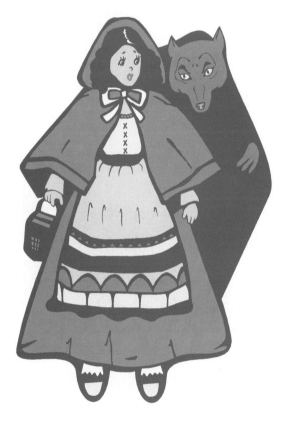

✓ **Apply contrasting color or tape to the edge of steps.**

✓ **Use telephones, clocks with extra large numbers.**

✓ **Use night lights.**

✓ **Use bright colors (avoid the use of blues and greens).**

✓ **Do not rearrange furniture (keep furniture in a familiar arrangement).**

163

✓ **Use lamps that do not throw a glare.**

✓ **Pause when going from a room with no light to a room with bright light and vice versa.**

✓ **Keep clutter off the floor.**

✓ **Keep a working flashlight at the bedside.**

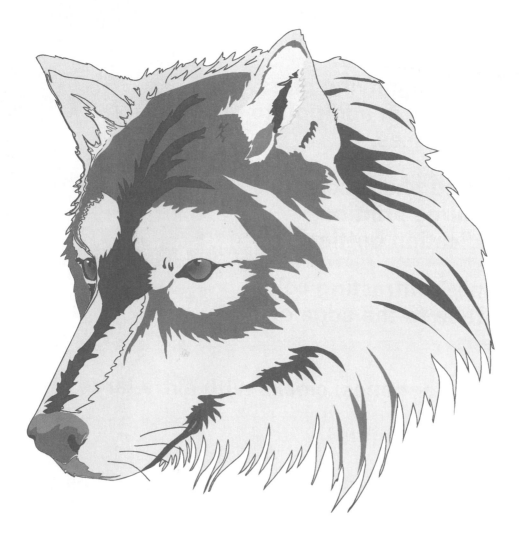

GRANNY, THE GLASSES, AND THE BIG, BAD WOLF

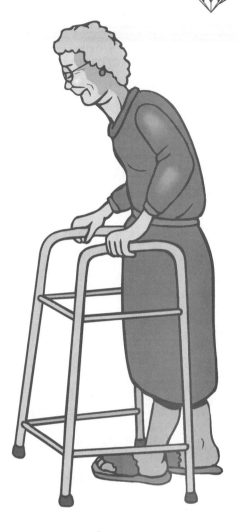

As the mean old bad wolf
paid a visit one morn,
Granny needed her glasses
that she always had worn.

She looked her house over.
She looked high and low.
Since she couldn't find her glasses
she told the stranger to go.

But he didn't leave;
he cried "I'm a little girl."
Without her magnifying glass
the wolf's ears looked like curls.

Granny asked the girl in,
Then poor Granny said,
"May I hang up your coat?"
The wolf nodded his head.

The glare from the lamp
had Granny confused.
She kept trying to see him,
the bad wolf was amused.

Granny began to get suspicious
when the wolf cried, "My head!"
Granny told the little sick girl,
"Go rest in my bed."

Her pharmacist, Tommy
was just as smart as could be.

165

He used extra large labels
so Granny could see.

She went to the cupboard;
the pills she did see.
"Here are two pills for you,"
"And two are for me."

The wolf feel asleep
and rested soundly in bed,
And awoke just as Granny
put the cape over his head.

In her sweet, granny voice
she said, "our heads ache no more.
Since we both now feel better,
let me show you the door."

As she pushed the wolf out
she found her glasses on the floor.
She called to the woodcutter
whom she now could see from the door.

She cried to the woodcutter
"That's a wolf, that's no girl."
Now Granny could see plainly
those were ears, those weren't curls.

The last thing Granny saw
was the flash of the chase,
as she washed up her glasses
and put them right on her face.

She said then and there
"I'll be more careful next time."
Be visually safe . . .
That's the moral to this rhyme.

—Gaye Ragland

166

CURLS or GIRL: Can You Tell The Difference?

· ·

1. What did Granny lose?

2. What could Granny have done differently to have kept from losing them?

3. What could Granny have used to see the wolf up close?

4. How did the pharmacist help Granny?

5. What did the lamp do to Granny's vision?

6. When Granny found her glasses, what did she do before she put them on?

7. Where do you store your glasses? Do you store them in the same place when you are not wearing them?

8. Do you clean your glasses regularly? How often?

9. Do you keep a night light on at night?

10. Do you pause when going to and from rooms with varying amounts of light?

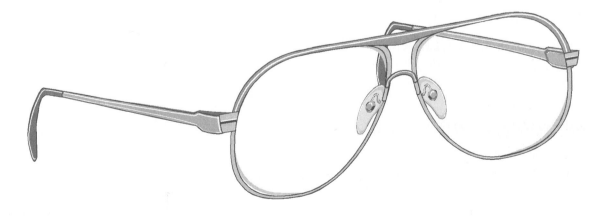

167

NUMBERS UP

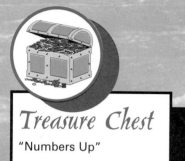

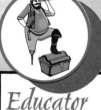

Treasure Chest

"Numbers Up"

Patients local telephone directory

Tape or tacks

Pen or pencil with an eraser

Educator Insights

"911" is **not** the emergency medical services access number in all areas. Be careful to list the correct local EMS phone number.

PREPARATION

1. Copy "Numbers Up" (both pages).
2. If the patient does not have one, obtain a telephone directory of listings in the patient's locale.
3. Make sure the patient has a pen or pencil with an eraser.

IMPLEMENTATION

1. Using the correct local emergency telephone numbers, complete "Numbers Up."
2. Ask the patient and/or caregiver to suggest where to post the numbers.
3. Assist the patient and/or caregiver to post "Numbers Up." Do not adhere lists to wallpaper or freshly painted walls.

By: Nancy Hollis, MSN, RN

NUMBERS UP

Keep the following numbers posted within full view.

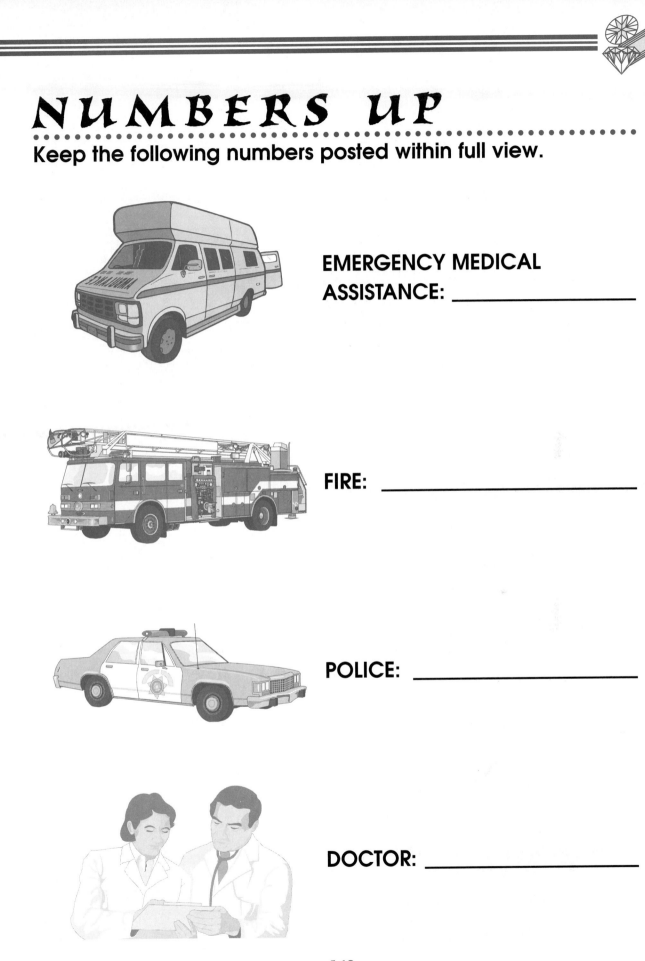

EMERGENCY MEDICAL
ASSISTANCE: _____

FIRE: _____

POLICE: _____

DOCTOR: _____

169

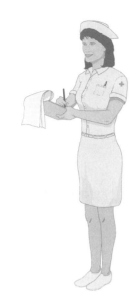

NURSE: _____

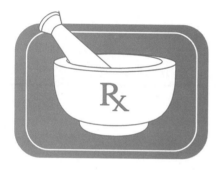

DRUG STORE: _____

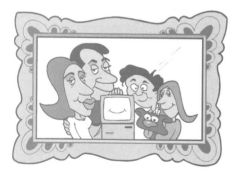

**NEAREST FAMILY
MEMBER:** _____

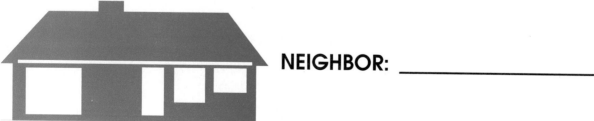

NEIGHBOR: _____

170

FALL CUT-OUT

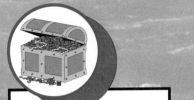

Treasure Chest

"Fall Cut-Out"

Scissors (blunt-end type)

2 pieces of brightly colored ribbon, each 3 inches long (optional)

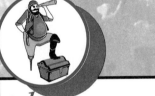

Educator Insights

You may tape (paper tape will do) two pieces of brightly colored ribbon to the back of the center block "No Falls for Me." Now tape the ribbon to the patient's shirt.

PREPARATION

1. Make two copies of "Fall Cut-Out." The patient will cut one copy, and an uncut copy should remain in the patient's home.

IMPLEMENTATION

1. Discuss with the patient the risks and effects of falling.
2. Have the patient cut away each square with blunt-end scissors as you discuss each square with him.
3. Discuss and cut away squares around outer perimeter first.
4. When all outer squares are cut, the patient is left with "No Falls for Me."
5. Post "No Falls for Me" on the bathroom mirror as a reminder for the patient to practice "Fall Prevention."
6. Leave uncut "Fall Cut-Out" with the patient.

By: Gaye Ragland, RN, BSN

171

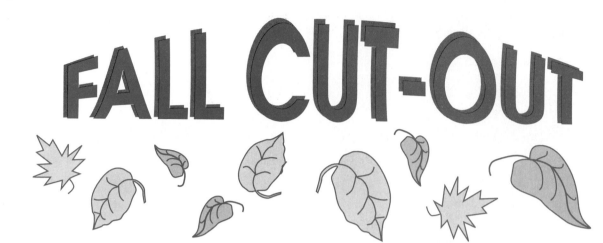

FALL CUT-OUT

Hold on to grab bars	Keep clutter off floor	Keep tissue off floor	Look at steps before going up or down	Wait for help to change high light bulbs	Get help if dizzy
Put non-skid mat or decals in tub or shower	Get puddles up quickly	Use walker, cane or other such devices properly	Hold to handrails on stairs or steps	Be careful of small pets	Watch for buckles in rugs
Keep night light on at night	Wear shoes with non-skid soles	**NO FALLS FOR ME**		Do not walk in sock/ stocking feet	Do not hurry to phone (or door); let caller wait
Keep cords off floor and out of path	Do not wear pants or robes too long			Keep newspaper off floor	Be careful walking in unfamiliar places
Keep phone within reach from floor	Stand up slowly	Get help on days you don't feel well	Be alert for icy build-up	Keep shoe laces tied	Look around before you walk
Keep hallways well lit	Hold on to something when rising	Do not climb on anything	Have loose handrails tightened	Do not use throw rugs/mats	Inspect home for hazards

172

HOW SAFE IS YOUR HOME?

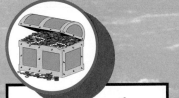

Treasure Chest

"How Safe Is Your Home?"

"Safety 'To Do' List"

Pen or pencil with an eraser

Educator Insights

Make all possible corrections as you make walking tour (i.e., cords on floor, clutter on floor, or safely replacing burned-out bulbs, if possible).

PREPARATION

1. Copy "How Safe Is Your Home?"
2. Allow time for a "walking tour" of the home with the patient and/or caregiver. Be prepared to complete the "Safety 'To Do' List."
3. Make sure the patient has a pen or pencil with an eraser.

IMPLEMENTATION

1. Ask the patient the questions on "How Safe Is Your Home?" question sheet.
2. Make notes on the questionnaire, if necessary.
3. When finished make a walking tour of the home. At this time, fill in the "Safety 'To Do' List."
4. Correct any safety hazards that you can, list those that need expert or outside help.
5. Call for immediate help if you find emergency hazards.
6. Leave all material in the patient's home.
7. Leave "Safety 'To Do' List" in an obvious place as a reminder to the patient and others who may offer to help.

By: Gaye Ragland, RN, BSN

HOW SAFE IS YOUR HOME?

INSTRUCTIONS: Answer each of the questions below.

1. Are all runners, carpets, mats, and throw rugs slip-resistant?

2. Are extension cords, lamp cords, and telephone cords out of the path of traffic?

3. Is any furniture resting on cords that could damage the cord creating shock and fire hazards?

4. Are there any cords in your house attached to the wall or baseboard (with staples, nails, or tacks) that could damage the cord creating a fire hazard?

5. Are you aware of any electrical cords in your home that are frayed or cracked?

6. Do you have any extension cords carrying more than the electrical load that they are approved to carry?

7. Are the following emergency numbers posted near the telephone for quick and easy access:

Police	Fire	Ambulance
Physician	Nurse	Hospital
Poison Control	Nearest Neighbor	Next of Kin

8. Do you have a telephone which you could get to in the event you should fall and become unable to stand and reach a wall phone?

9. Is there at least one smoke detector on each floor of your home?

10. Are smoke detectors in proper working order with fresh batteries?

11. Do any switches or electrical outlets in your home feel warm to the touch?

174

12. Are light bulbs the proper size for the fixture?

13. Do all electrical outlets have switches and cover plates?

14. Are all plugs being used in the proper type of outlet, or do they at least have the proper adapter (for example, are 3 prong plugs in 3 hole outlets, etc.)?

15. Are small heaters and stoves out of the passageway and away from draperies, rugs, furniture, etc.?

16. Do you understand the correct way your heater works? To the best of your knowledge, is it installed according to the installation instructions?

17. Can you explain how you would get out of or leave the house in the event of fire (the different routes of evacuation from different areas of your home supposing the fire was located in different rooms)?

18. Is the area nearest your stove free from electrical cords, throw rugs, mats, dish towels, and other items that could catch fire from your range?

19. Do you wear clothing with close fitting sleeves or short sleeves when you are cooking (to prevent the garment sleeve from coming in contact with heat or flames)?

20. Is your kitchen well-lighted?

21. Do you climb on boxes, furniture, or other household items to change bulbs or to reach high places, or do you wait for someone to help you?

22. Are hallways in your home well-lighted?

23. Is medication in your home out of the reach of children or grandchildren?

24. Do you keep all medication either in the original labeled bottle or in a container that is clearly marked?

25. Do you dispose of outdated medications properly?

26. Does your bathtub (or shower) have a non-skid mat?

27. Do you have grab bars near your tub, shower, and toilet? Are they fastened securely?

28. Do you keep clutter picked up off the floor?

29. Is the path clear around the bed and to the bathroom?

30. Is the water temperature of your hot water heater set at "low" or 120 degrees?

31. Do you always check the water temperature with your hand before you get into the tub?

32. Do you keep small electrical appliances unplugged when not in use?

33. Can you reach a light from the bed?

34. Can you reach a telephone from the bed?

35. Are there ash trays, smoking materials, coffee pots, or any fire hazard near the bed?

36. Do you follow manufacturer's instructions for use of electric blankets (not tucking in the sides, not placing anything on top, and keeping temperature regulated low enough to prevent a burn)?

37. Do you always keep the temperature of your heating pad at a low setting?

38. Do you always turn the heating pad off before going to bed?

39. Can you turn lights on without first having to walk through areas that are dark?

40. Do you keep an operating flashlight handy?

41. Do you have a battery powered radio and a supply of fresh batteries?

42. Are containers of volatile liquids tightly capped?

43. Are gasoline, paints, solvents, or other products that give off vapors stored away from ignition sources?

44. Are handrails securely attached on the sides of stairways?

45. Do your steps allow secure footing?

46. Is the carpeting free from buckles that could cause you to trip?

47. Do handrails run from the top to the bottom of your steps?

48. Are all steps or stairways well-lighted?

49. Do you always leave a night light on at night?

50. Do you agree to be "safety minded" and periodically recheck your home for safety hazards?

ADAPTED FROM: *Safety For Older Consumers Home Safety Checklist* booklet produced by U.S. Consumer Product Safety Commission, Washington, D.C.

SAFETY "TO DO" LIST

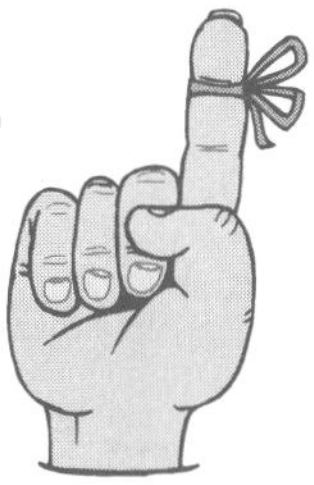

ITEM 1: _____

_____ Completed? check here ☐

ITEM 2: _____

_____ Completed? check here ☐

ITEM 3: _____

_____ Completed? check here ☐

ITEM 4: _____

_____ Completed? check here ☐

ITEM 5: _____

_____ Completed? check here ☐

ITEM 6: _____

_____ Completed? check here ☐

ITEM 7: _____

_____ Completed? check here ☐

SAFETY RHYMES AND REASONS

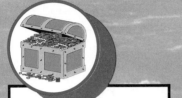

PATIENT SAFETY

Treasure Chest

"Notes On Safety"

"Safety Rhymes and Reasons"

Big brimmed hat or wire-rimmed glasses (optional)

Pen or pencil with an eraser

Educator Insights

If desired, you may wear funny hat and/or glasses or you may choose to read (to selected patients) with funny voices and much, much expression prior to a serious examination of the content.

PREPARATION

1. Review and copy "Notes On Safety."
2. Copy "Safety Rhymes and Reasons."
3. Make sure the patient has a pen or pencil with an eraser.

IMPLEMENTATION

1. Read "Notes On Safety" with the patient.
2. Explain to the patient that you will read "Safety Rhymes and Reasons."
3. Read "Safety Rhymes and Reasons."
4. After the initial reading, go through each section and talk about the implications for safety.
5. Leave "Safety Rhymes and Reasons" with the patient.

By: Gaye Ragland, RN, BSN

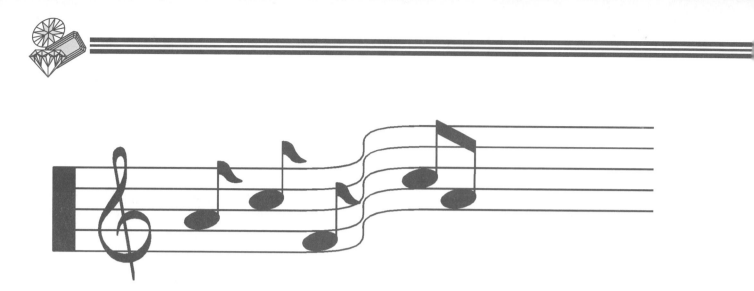

NOTES ON SAFETY

Many senior citizens are treated each year in emergency rooms for accidents that could have been easily prevented. After an accident happens, it is often said, "I knew better than to have done that" or "I just don't know what came over me." Risk-taking causes accidents and can result in pain, disability, risk to other people, and even death.

Many injuries that result from accidents are caused by hazards that could have been easily prevented. Many of those same hazards could have been fixed with little or no effort at all. Are there accident hazards in your home? Keep these notes and the notes to follow. Review them now. Save them to review in the future.

SAFETY RHYMES AND REASONS

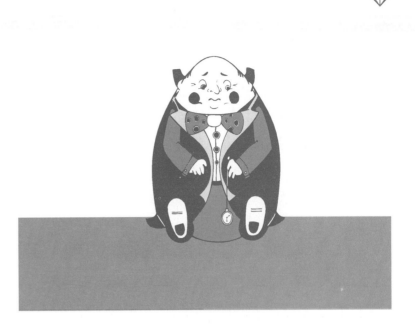

THERE WAS AN OLD WOMAN WHO TRIPPED ON A SHOE.
SHE HAD SO MANY BROKEN BONES SHE DIDN'T KNOW WHAT TO DO.
AS SHE LAY ON THE FLOOR AND HOPED SOMEONE WOULD CALL,
SHE REGRETTED CHANGING THE LIGHT BULB WHICH CAUSED HER TO FALL.

BIG 'OL MACK MOURNER, HE SAT IN THE CORNER
FROM A FRAYED CORD HE WATCHED A SPARK FLY.
HE STUCK IN HIS THUMB AND THAT REALLY WAS DUMB
ELECTRICAL ACCIDENTS CAUSE PEOPLE TO DIE.

SUE AND BILL WENT DOWN THE HILL
TO FETCH SOME WATER FOR THEIR HOMES.
THE HILL HAD ICED; THEY DIDN'T KNOW
NOW EACH OF THEM HAS BROKEN BONES.

TED, TED HAS QUITE A HARD HEAD.
HOW WELL DO YOUR HOUSE NUMBERS SHOW?
WITH FADED PAINT AND NO PORCH LIGHT
EMERGENCY SERVICES WOULD NOT KNOW WHERE TO GO.

181

MARY HAD AN EMERGENCY CARD

THE CARD WAS WHITE AS SNOW.

AND EVERY TRIP THAT MARY TOOK

THE CARD WAS SURE TO GO.

SO IF MARY SHOULD BECOME SUDDENLY ILL

THE CARD WOULD TELL THE TALE,

OF WHO MARY WAS AND WHO SHOULD BE CALLED

SO MARY COULD GET HELP TO GET WELL.

LITTLE MISTER PUFF IT

LIKED HAVING TO HUFF IT,

SO HE KEPT SMOKING THOSE DANGEROUS WEEDS,

NOT ONLY IS THE HABIT BAD FOR HIS HEALTH

BUT CAN BE A FIRE HAZARD, IF CARELESS, INDEED.

BE SURE THAT YOU NEVER, EVER LIGHT UP IN BED

OR SMOKE IF THERE IS OXYGEN NEARBY.

AND WHEN YOU PUT IT OUT, MAKE SURE IT IS OUT,

SMOKING ACCIDENTS CAUSE PEOPLE TO CRY.

ANNIE WAS NIMBLE, ANNIE WAS QUICK

TO CALL FOR HELP WHEN SHE GOT SICK.

SHE KEPT THE NUMBERS BY HER PHONE

SO HER NEED FOR HELP COULD BE QUICKLY MADE KNOWN.

LITTLE BO JO NEARLY LOST HIS HOUSE

AND DIDN'T KNOW WHERE IT COULD BE.

HE NEVER PAID HEED TO BAD WEATHER REPORTS

AND COULD HAVE BEEN BLOWN FAR AWAY SO YOU SEE.

SO NOW LITTLE BO JO KEEPS A RADIO CLOSE
AND LISTENS ON BAD, STORMY DAYS.
HE KNOWS IF IT'S COLD, HE KNOWS IF IT'S HOT,
BEING ALERT, BO JO SAYS, 'REALLY PAYS!'

BAKE-A-CAKE, BAKE-A-CAKE, LIKE NO GRANNY CAN;
SHE'S BAKING AND COOKING JUST AS FAST AS SHE CAN.
SHE'S NOW VERY TIRED AND RETIRES TO THE LOFT.
IT IS VERY IMPORTANT THAT GRANNY'S STOVE IS TURNED OFF.

WITH ALL OF THESE RHYMES TO HELP YOU, YOU SEE,
YOU WILL SURELY REMEMBER TO BE AS CAREFUL AS CAN BE.
KEEP YOUR MIND ON SAFE HABITS WHETHER AT HOME OR AWAY.
KEEP YOUR HEAD UP AND EYES OPEN EACH NIGHT AND EACH DAY.

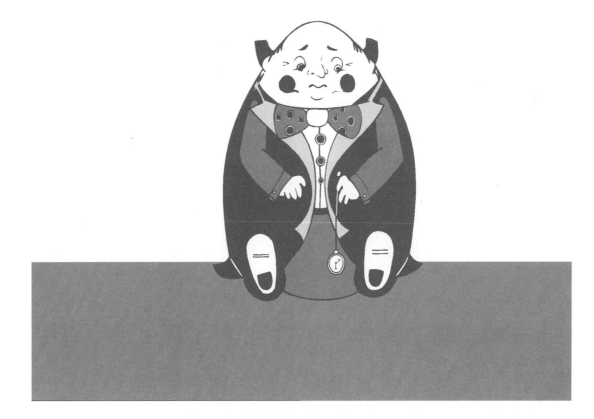

AGREEMENT AND CERTIFICATE FOR SAFETY

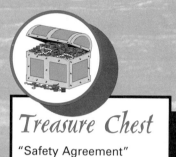

Treasure Chest

"Safety Agreement"

"Safety Certificate"

Black ink pen

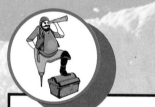

Educator Insights

Be sure the patient does not perceive this agreement to be a binding, legal contract of any nature.

PREPARATION

1. Copy "Safety Agreement."
2. Copy "Safety Certificate."
3. Use "How Safe Is Your Home" and other selected safety teaching tools before signing the "Safety Agreement" and before awarding the "Safety Certificate."

IMPLEMENTATION

1. Continue to emphasize home safety and fall prevention, encourage the patient to assume the responsibility for minimizing or eliminating hazards and to practice fall prevention.
2. Read and discuss the "Safety Agreement" with the patient. If the patient agrees, fill in the name blank at the top and the date and signature blanks at the bottom.
3. As a reward for the efforts made to "safety-proof" the home and for the commitment to continue to practice safety and fall prevention, complete the "Safety Certificate" and present it to the patient.
4. Leave the completed copy in the patient's home.

By: Gaye Ragland, RN, BSN

SAFETY AGREEMENT

DIRECTIONS: Read and sign.

I, _____, agree to live by good safety practices as follows:

Henceforth, I will not climb on stools, chairs, or furniture to get higher than the ground and,

Henceforth, I will keep clutter off the floor and electrical cords removed from my path and from around my bed and,

Henceforth, I will walk only in well-lighted areas and,

Henceforth, I will look at steps before I use them and,

Henceforth, I will hold onto handrails if they are available and,

Henceforth, I will use my walker, crutches, or cane as ordered or approved by my doctor and,

Henceforth, I will check my smoke detectors periodically and keep them in good working order and,

Henceforth, I will keep my eyes open and my head up, being alert to safety risks and hazards and,

Henceforth, I will ask for help when needed to assure my personal and household safety.

This the _____ day of _____

Signed by _____

Caregiver _____

185

Safety Certificate

AWARDED TO

_____

For Participation In "Home Safety" Training Program Taught by

_____
Presented By

_____
Date

UP . . . UP . . . AND DELAY

Treasure Chest

"Up . . . Up . . . and Delay"

"Rules To Rise By"

2 Helium-filled balloons with strings

Pen or pencil with an eraser

Educator Insights

Help the patient watch the balloons from the door or window if unable to go outside. This exercise can be done with only one balloon.

PREPARATION

1. Make a copy of "Up . . . Up . . . and Delay."
2. Make a copy of "Rules To Rise By."
3. Obtain two helium-filled balloons.
4. Make sure the patient has a pen or pencil with an eraser.

IMPLEMENTATION

1. Initiate discussion about past episodes of feeling dizzy or faint after quickly moving from a sitting to a standing position. (Many patients can relate to this when reminded of working in a garden on a hot, summer day.)
2. Using "Up . . . Up . . . and Delay" teach the cause and effects of orthostatic hypotension (i.e., low blood pressure when standing).
3. If the patient is able, step outside into an area free of power lines or trees.
4. As both you and the patient release your balloons, talk about rising very slowly.
5. Hold the patient securely to prevent a fall, as you and the patient watch the balloons.
6. If the patient is unable to go outdoors, you may modify this activity using one balloon and watching it float to the ceiling.
7. Give the patient "Rules To Rise By."
8. After discussing "Rules To Rise By," assist the patient, if necessary, to fill in the blanks and solve the riddle at the bottom of the page.
9. Leave "Up . . . Up . . . and Delay" with the patient.

By: Gaye Ragland, RN, BSN

187

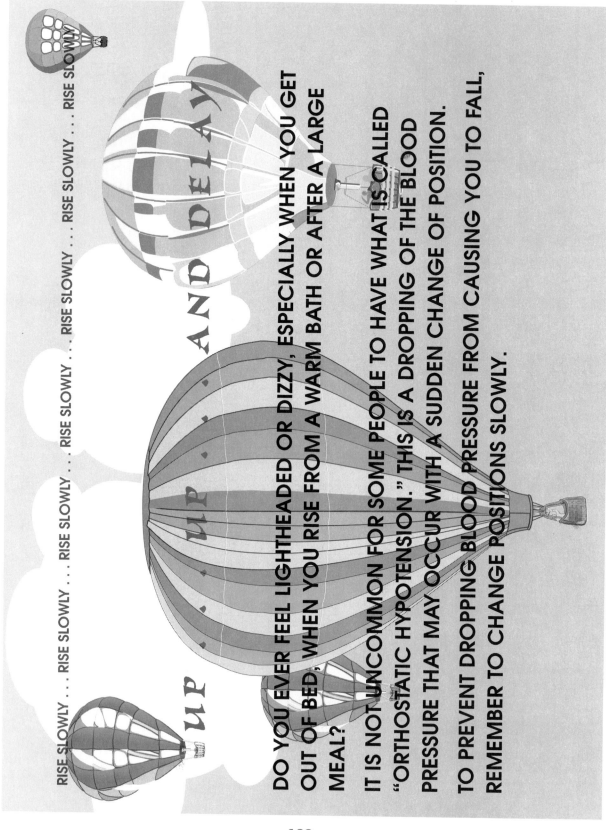

RISE SLOWLY . . . RISE SLOWLY . . . RISE SLOWLY . . . RISE SLOWLY . . . RISE SLOWLY . . . RISE SLOWLY

UP . . . UP . . . AND AWAY

DO YOU EVER FEEL LIGHTHEADED OR DIZZY, ESPECIALLY WHEN YOU GET OUT OF BED, WHEN YOU RISE FROM A WARM BATH OR AFTER A LARGE MEAL?

IT IS NOT UNCOMMON FOR SOME PEOPLE TO HAVE WHAT IS CALLED "ORTHOSTATIC HYPOTENSION." THIS IS A DROPPING OF THE BLOOD PRESSURE THAT MAY OCCUR WITH A SUDDEN CHANGE OF POSITION.

TO PREVENT DROPPING BLOOD PRESSURE FROM CAUSING YOU TO FALL, REMEMBER TO CHANGE POSITIONS SLOWLY.

188

Rules to Rise By

Directions: Put the missing letters in the blanks below.

1. SIT ON THE SIDE OF THE __ED FOR SEVERAL MINUTES BEFORE MOVING INTO A STANDING POSITION.

2. DO NOT ST__ND FOR LONG PERIODS OF TIME.

3. CHANGE POSITIONS S__OW__Y.

4. H__LD ON TO SOMEONE OR SOMETHING SECURE AS YOU SL__WLY STAND.

5. WHEN RISING AFTER LYING FOR A LO__G PERIOD OF TIME, CALL FOR HELP, IF NEEDED.

Clue: It is a fun but slow moving way to travel.

_ _ _ _ _ _ _ _   (LONBLOA)

189

Rules to Rise By

Answer Key

1. SIT ON THE SIDE OF THE BED FOR SEVERAL MINUTES BEFORE MOVING INTO A STANDING POSITION.

2. DO NOT STAND FOR LONG PERIODS OF TIME.

3. CHANGE POSITIONS SLOWLY.

4. HOLD TO SOMEONE OR SOMETHING SECURE AS YOU SLOWLY STAND.

5. WHEN RISING AFTER LYING FOR A LONG PERIOD OF TIME, CALL FOR HELP, IF NEEDED.

Clue: It is a fun but slow moving way to travel.

B A L L O O N

DON'T ASPIRATE WHAT YOU JUST ATE

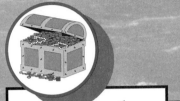

ASPIRATION

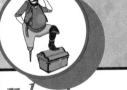

Treasure Chest

"Don't Aspirate What You Just Ate"

"More Tips for Aspiration Prevention"

"Heads Up"

Pen or pencil with an eraser

Educator Insights

Be sure to include family members as you teach aspiration prevention.

PREPARATION

1. Review and copy "Don't Aspirate What You Just Ate" and "More Tips for Aspiration Prevention."
2. Review and copy "Heads Up."
3. Make sure the patient has a pen or pencil with an eraser.

IMPLEMENTATION

1. Review "Don't Aspirate What You Just Ate" and "More Tips for Aspiration Prevention" with the patient and/or caregiver.
2. On "Heads Up" from point "X" on the mattresses, draw a single line to form the proper angle of elevation (30°, 45°, etc.) of the head of the bed as ordered by the patient's doctor.
3. Leave "Don't Aspirate What You Just Ate," "More Tips for Aspiration Prevention," and "Heads Up" with the caregiver.

By: Gaye Ragland, RN, BSN

DON'T ASPIRATE *What* **you** JUST ATE

The term aspiration means . . . "to draw material such as saliva, mucus, or food particles into the lungs from the mouth." This can happen when the cough or gag reflex is delayed or is not strong enough to push the fluid upward and into the mouth. It can happen to an unconscious patient. It can happen to a weak, frail patient who does not have the strength to cough. It can happen to a patient who is unable to move about and is lying on his/her back.

To lessen the risk of aspiration, raise the head of the bed 30 to 45 degrees during meals and for at least one hour after meals, if possible (with doctor's approval). If the patient is able to be up and out of the bed for meals and for part of the day, have the patient remain up for 2 to 3 hours after eating. This will allow time for the food to begin to leave the stomach. The food will be less likely to be vomited and aspirated back into the lungs. Ask the doctor or nurse if the patient can sit up in bed. If so, sit the patient up in bed and support the patient's sides with pillows.

More Tips for Aspiration Prevention

✗ Remind the patient to take small bites.

✗ Remind the patient to chew the food and swallow after each bite.

✗ Watch for food held in the mouth. Remind the patient not to hold food in his mouth.

✗ Encourage the patient to rest before mealtime. The risk is greater if the patient is tired.

✗ If the patient has dentures, put them in place before meals.

✗ Be sure the patient's dentures fit properly.

✗ Stay with the patient during mealtime.

✗ Remind confused patients to chew and swallow each bite.

✗ Allow the patient adequate time to eat. Do not rush the patient.

Heads Up

Directions: Ask the nurse or doctor to draw the backrest to the mattresses below to show how high the patient should sit up in bed to eat.

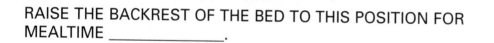

RAISE THE BACKREST OF THE BED TO THIS POSITION FOR MEALTIME _____.

LEAVE THE BACKREST OF THE BED IN THIS POSITION FOR _____ HOURS AFTER MEALS

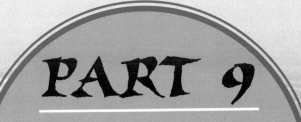

PART 9

Instant Treasures for Specific Diseases

ALZHEIMER'S FROM "A" TO "Z"

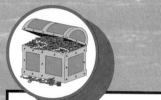

Treasure Chest

"Alzheimer's from 'A' to 'Z'"

"Say The Word"

"Daily Care Tips"

"Alzheimer's Word Search"

"Alzheimer's Word Search" answer key

Pen or pencil with an eraser

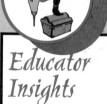

Educator Insights

The caregivers of Alzheimer patients often become drained. Refer to "Caregiver Storm Warning" to assess the caregiver's stress, if necessary.

PREPARATION

1. Copy and review "Alzheimer's from 'A' to 'Z'."
2. Copy and review "Say the Word."
3. Copy and review "Daily Care Tips."
4. Copy "Alzheimer's Word Search."
5. Copy "Alzheimer's Word Search" answer key.
6. Make sure the caregiver has a pen or pencil with an eraser.
7. Provide local telephone numbers for support groups and community resources.

IMPLEMENTATION

1. Discuss "Alzheimer's from 'A' to 'Z'" with the caregiver. Point out the highlighted words and explain that those words are hidden in the puzzle, "Alzheimer's Word Search."
2. Discuss the "Say the Word" sheet. Teach the caregiver to pronounce "Alzheimer's."
3. Review the "Daily Care Tips" teaching sheet.
4. Ask the caregiver to complete the word search puzzle.
5. Check the answers when the caregiver is finished.
6. Leave "Alzheimer's from 'A' to 'Z'" with the caregiver.

By: Billie Phillips, MSN, RN, and
Bonnie Davis, RN, DNS

Alzheimer's from "A" to "Z"

Alzheimer's is a **progressive,** irreversible disease of the **brain.** Progressive means that the signs and symptoms worsen as the disease continues. The brain is affected causing loss of **memory,** thinking, and judgement. Although Alzheimer's disease is more common in persons over **65** years of age, it does occur in middle-aged persons. It affects more women than men. Alzheimer's is a form of **dementia.**

There is no cure for Alzheimer's, which is why it is called irreversible. There is no one test to determine that someone has the disease. The doctor rules out other possible diseases and then evaluates the signs and symptoms the patient has.

Symptoms vary, but Alzheimer's disease is usually defined by **three stages.**

STAGE ONE lasts from two to four years and may include the following symptoms:

- ▶ **Apathy:** losing interest in activities and life
- ▶ Being confused about place and time
- ▶ Making poor judgements
- ▶ Forgeting to pay bills

- ▶ Becoming concerned about self
- ▶ Becoming **forgetful,** hiding things, and becoming **angry** when the hiding place cannot be remembered
- ▶ Believing possessions have been stolen
- ▶ Driving somewhere and forgetting the destination
- ▶ No longer caring about appearance: may not bathe or change clothes

STAGE TWO may last from two to ten years and may include the following symptoms:

- ▶ **Restlessness,** especially in the late afternoon; this is called **sundowning**
- ▶ Being unable to recognize family and/or friends
- ▶ **Suspiciousness:** thinking they are going to be harmed
- ▶ Repeating the same sentence over and over
- ▶ Becoming more **immobile:** has trouble walking and sitting
- ▶ **Rummaging** and **hoarding:** spending hours going through drawers and closets, sorting silverware or socks
- ▶ **Crying,** becoming **combative** when approached
- ▶ **Clinging** to the caregiver
- ▶ **Wandering,** causing a **safety** problem
- ▶ **Insomnia:** being unable to sleep because sleep patterns are interrupted
- ▶ Having **delusions** about themselves and those around them
- ▶ Reliving prior life events

STAGE THREE usually lasts from one to three years and may include the following symptoms:

- ▶ Weight loss; **nutrition,** however may be adequate
- ▶ Being unable to care for self
- ▶ Having no control over bowel and bladder
- ▶ Being unable to communicate with words

Care of the person with Alzheimer's disease is emotionally and physically exhausting for the caregiver. Support groups offer understanding and sharing of experiences that may provide comfort.

Say the Word

("Alzheimer's," That Is!)

 Properly pronounce "ALZHEIMER'S" (Pronounced Altz-hi-merz).

 Repeat the word aloud.

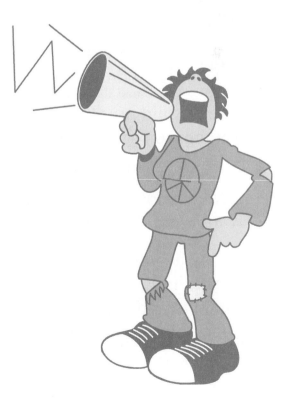

✗ Word associate the word with the word "WALTZ (the dance).

✗ Say: "WALTZ-HI-MERS"

✗ Now, drop the "W" and say:

"ALZHEIMER'S"

✗ Repeat the word three times.

Daily Care Tips

FOR THE ALZHEIMER'S PATIENT

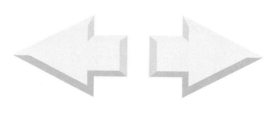

1. Use large calendars, clocks, newspapers that show the date.

2. Do not quiz the patient or ask the patient to remember or think.

3. Talk with the patient about happy times in the past.

4. Place signs on the doors and drawers to show their use.

5. Have a bracelet made that is not easily removed. Include the patient's name, address, telephone number, and "memory loss."

6. Remove knobs from stove when not in use.

7. Place a bell on outside door so you can hear when the patient goes outside during the day.

8. Place "child proof" knobs on the doors at night. These can be purchased at hardware stores.

9. Go with the patient on walks to promote interest in living. This also promotes exercise and sleep and prevents restless wandering.

10. Put away valuables such as rings and money that the patient might "hide" and forget. Limit hiding places by locking some cabinets and closets. Check wastebaskets before emptying them. Keep spare keys and glasses in a safe place.

11. Go by the same daily schedule as much as possible.

12. If the patient's actions are inappropriate, distract the patient. Do not confront the patient.

13. If the patient shows poor judgement or talks about things as they were long ago, answer the "feeling" rather than correcting the fact. Example: "I want to go home." (When they are at home). Say, "Yes, I know you want to go home" (to the way things used to be).

14. If the patient is rude or demanding to friends or strangers, privately explain the patient's condition.

15. Give the patient simple tasks he/she is able to do with guidance. Examples: folding clothes, sweeping, watering plants.

16. Guide grooming and dressing with simple instructions given one step at a time.

17. Include the patient in family events. Be careful not to over-stimulate.

18. If the patient is messy or plays with food, consider using a bowl rather than a plate, giving only one food at a time, using "finger" foods, cutting meats in bite sizes, using a plastic apron.

19. Notify neighbors of the patient's condition if there is a chance the patient may wander away.

20. Notify the local law enforcement agency of the patient's condition if there is a chance the patient may wander away.

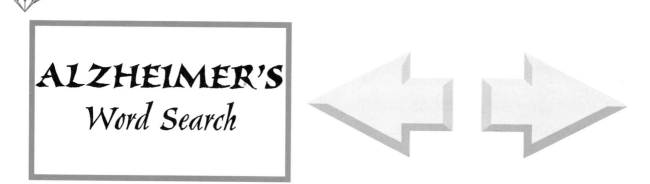

ALZHEIMER'S
Word Search

Directions: Find the hidden words taken from **"Alzheimer's from 'A to Z.'"**

Remember: The words can be forward, backward, up and down, and diagonal.

C	R	N	S	D	E	M	E	N	T	I	A	M	E	R	O	P	C
A	L	Z	H	E	I	M	E	R	S	K	Y	C	T	U	O	C	D
R	B	G	O	F	L	A	S	M	P	A	T	O	L	M	D	L	P
E	N	B	A	P	A	T	H	Y	W	S	X	M	C	M	F	I	E
G	A	N	R	B	M	X	I	Z	T	S	W	B	R	A	I	N	S
I	O	K	D	A	L	Q	A	S	D	P	H	A	U	G	Y	G	O
V	W	S	I	X	R	F	V	T	G	R	B	T	Y	I	H	I	I
E	K	I	N	U	T	R	I	T	I	O	N	I	J	N	U	N	U
R	Q	A	G	Z	W	E	S	X	E	G	D	V	C	G	R	G	Y
K	I	M	J	U	N	S	H	Y	B	R	G	E	S	T	V	F	T
O	L	P	Z	X	C	T	V	B	N	E	M	L	U	K	J	H	G
P	O	I	U	Y	T	L	R	E	W	S	Q	A	N	S	W	D	F
I	M	M	O	B	I	L	E	H	J	S	K	L	D	J	A	H	G
G	F	D	S	A	Z	S	X	C	V	I	N	S	O	M	N	I	A
J	S	T	A	G	E	S	U	K	I	V	O	L	W	M	D	N	B
W	A	S	E	D	F	T	G	H	Y	E	U	A	N	G	E	R	M
X	F	O	R	G	E	T	F	U	L	V	B	D	I	H	R	N	E
W	E	F	T	Y	H	J	I	K	L	O	N	G	N	H	I	S	M
C	T	G	U	H	Y	R	G	C	R	Y	I	N	G	R	N	A	O
R	Y	E	D	C	T	G	B	Y	H	N	U	J	M	K	G	I	R
D	E	L	U	S	I	O	N	S	U	J	M	K	I	L	O	P	Y
W	S	C	S	U	S	P	I	C	I	O	U	S	N	E	S	S	D

WORDS

Alzheimer's
Apathy
Brain
Caregiver
Combative
Crying

Delusions
Dementia
Forgetful
Immobile
Insomnia
Memory

Nutrition
Progressive
Role
Rummaging
Safety
Stages

Sundowning
Suspicious
Wandering

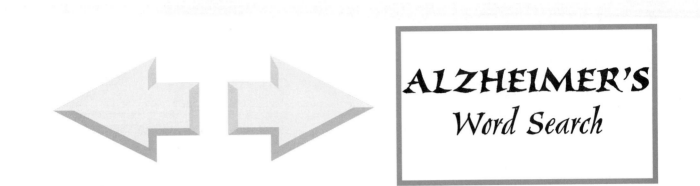

ALZHEIMER'S
Word Search

ANSWER KEY:

```
C R N S D E M E N T I A M E R O P C
A L Z H E I M E R S K Y C T U O C D
R B G O F L A S M P A T O L M D L P
E N B A P A T H Y W S X M C M F I E
G A N R B M X I Z T S W B R A I N S
I O K D A L Q A S D P H A U G Y G O
V W S I X R F V T G R B T Y I H I I
E K I N U T R I T I O N I J N U N U
R Q A G Z W E S X E G D V C G R G Y
K I M J U N S H Y B R G E S T V F T
O L P Z X C T V B N E M L U K J H G
P O I U Y T L R E W S Q A N S W D F
I M M O B I L E H J S K L D J A H G
G F D S A Z S X C V I N S O M N I A
J S T A G E S U K I V O L W M D N B
W A S E D F T G H Y E U A N G E R M
X F O R G E T F U L V B D I H R N E
W E F T Y H J I K L O N G N H I S M
C T G U H Y R G C R Y I N G R N A O
R Y E D C T G B Y H N U J M K G I R
D E L U S I O N S U J M K I L O P Y
W S C S U S P I C I O U S N E S S D
```

203

HANDLING HYPERTENSION

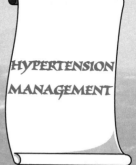

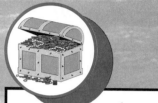

Treasure Chest

"It's High Time You Know About Hypertension"

"Risky Business"

"Handling Hypertension Instruction Sheet"

"Handling Hypertension" activity sheet

Pen or pencil with an eraser

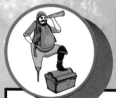

Educator Insights

You may **highlight** with a brightly colored marker any specific **problem area(s)** or those that will be the greatest challenge to the particular patient.

PREPARATION

1. Copy and review "It's High Time You Know About Hypertension" fact sheet.
2. Copy and review "Risky Business" fact sheet.
3. Copy and review "Handling Hypertension Instruction Sheet."
4. Copy the "Handling Hypertension" page for tracing.
5. Make sure the patient has a pen or pencil with an eraser.

IMPLEMENTATION

1. Use handouts "It's High Time You Know about Hypertension" and "Risky Business" to teach hypertension management and risk factors.
2. After teaching the patient about ways to control hypertension, have the patient trace both of their hands on the page titled "Handling Hypertension." You will have to trace the hands for some patients.
3. Assist the patient writing specific ways he or she will control their blood pressure.
4. Use the 10 ways to control hypertension listed on the "Handling Hypertension Instruction Sheet."
5. Leave "Handling Hypertension" with the patient.

By: Gaye Ragland, RN, BSN

204

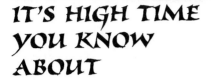

IT'S HIGH TIME YOU KNOW ABOUT

HYPERTENSION
(High Blood Pressure)

Similar to the way the water hydrant in your backyard pumps water through the garden hose, the heart pumps blood through your arteries. If your garden hose becomes twisted, preventing the flow of water through it, think of how the hose stretches in response to the added pressure. In a similar way, the walls of your healthy arteries stretch as the pressure from each beat of the heart forces blood through them. The arteries supply the much needed blood-containing oxygen to all the parts of your body. When the heart rests between heartbeats, the pressure goes down.

When your doctor or nurse checks your blood pressure, you will notice that two numbers are recorded. One of the numbers is written on top of a line and another number is written below the line. The one that is written first and on top is called the **"systolic"** pressure. It measures the pressure in your arteries that occurs when the heart is beating. The second number is called the **"diastolic"** pressure. It measures the pressure in the arteries that occurs while your heart is resting between beats.

205

Normal blood pressure falls within a range of numbers. The blood pressure can change from minute to minute, depending on what you are doing or how you are feeling. It can change if you are exercising. It can change if you are in pain. It can change if you are very worried. It can change when you change positions. It can even change while you are sleeping.

If your doctor or nurse finds your blood pressure to be high, your blood pressure will need to be checked again. It is usually recommended that it be checked a couple of more times at about the same time of day to determine if the elevation was a single incident or if you need to be on medication.

High blood pressure is sometimes called **"the silent killer."** Unless the blood pressure just happens to be checked, most people don't know that their blood pressure is elevated. If you know you have high blood pressure or if you have a family history of high blood pressure, it is important to have your pressure checked regularly.

The reason people have high blood pressure is not known in most cases. In cases where the cause is unknown, the patient is said to have "primary hypertension" or "essential hypertension." Even though the cause of high blood pressure may not be known, there **are** some specific factors (called risk factors) that make a person more prone to have high blood pressure.

To determine your risk factors read the following fact sheet called **"Risky Business."**

206

Risky Business

Determining Your Risk for High Blood Pressure

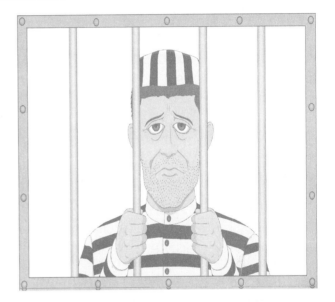

FAMILY HISTORY

If your parents or other close blood relatives have high blood pressure, there is an increased chance that you will have it, too.

Though the exact links of family members having high blood pressure are not clearly understood, it is known that high blood pressure tends to run in families. It is not certain whether those links are genetic or because family members tend to eat the same foods and live in similar environments.

MALE or FEMALE

Until they reach 60 years of age, men develop higher blood pressure and develop it at younger ages than women. Men also tend to have a greater risk than women of developing heart disease.

AGE

The older we get, the more likely we are to develop high blood pressure. This is because the older our arteries, the less flexible they become, usually due to the fatty build-up inside the walls. Because

207

older patients have been exposed to this risk factor for so long, they often have greater complications than younger patients.

ETHNIC GROUPS

High blood pressure occurs more frequently in blacks than in whites. High blood pressure tends to occur earlier and be more serious in blacks.

STRESS

It is felt that some psychological factors may influence the blood pressure. It is suggested that certain personality types as well as particularly stressful jobs have been linked to elevations of the blood pressure. However, it is difficult to measure exact amounts of stress and the way people handle it.

EXERCISE

Most people who do not exercise find that they easily gain extra weight. People who are physically active gain the benefits of both controlling their weight and decreasing body fat. Anyone starting an exercise program should check with their doctor.

ALCOHOL

The regular and heavy use of alcohol can increase a person's chances of developing high blood pressure.

SMOKING

The exact relationship between smoking and high blood pressure is not totally clear. What is clear is that smoking does increase the risk of heart disease and stroke. Smoking may make efforts to control your high blood pressure more difficult.

DIET

A high amount of salt intake has an effect on some people who have high blood pressure.

HANDLING HYPERTENSION
INSTRUCTION SHEET

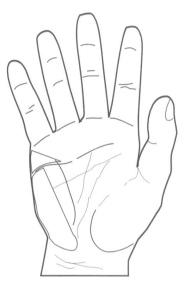

Trace your patient's hands on the page titled "Handling Hypertension" that follows. When finished tracing, discuss the ways to control hypertension that are listed below. As you discuss each topic, have the patient write the topic on one of the ten fingers. Talk about the ways the indivdual patient can make necessary lifestyle changes to gain better control of the hypertension.

1. Take your blood pressure medication as prescribed.
2. Don't smoke.
3. Get (or keep) weight within normal limits.
4. Be physically active within the limits prescribed by your doctor.
5. Reduce stress if possible.
6. Reduce salt intake. Stick to the diet prescribed by your doctor.
7. Have your blood pressure checked periodically.
8. Know the usual range for your blood pressure.
9. Have regular check-ups.
10. Limit alcohol intake according to your doctor's orders.

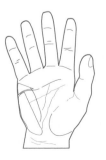

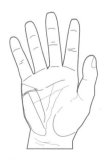

HANDLING HYPERTENSION

CONTROLLING HYPERTENSION CROSSWORD

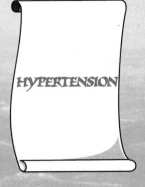

HYPERTENSION

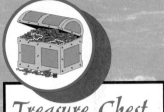

Treasure Chest

"Controlling Hypertension" crossword puzzle

"Controlling Hypertension" answer key

Pen or pencil with an eraser

Educator Insights

If the patient is unable to work the puzzle, consider working it together, repeating the information just one more time.

PREPARATION

1. Copy "Controlling Hypertension" crossword puzzle.
2. Copy the answer key to "Controlling Hypertension" crossword puzzle.
3. Make sure the patient has a pen or pencil with an eraser.

IMPLEMENTATION

1. Ask the patient to complete the crossword puzzle.
2. Explain that the answers to the puzzle can be found in the handouts "Risky Business" and "It's High Time You Know About Hypertension."
3. Check the patient's answers when the puzzle is completed or leave the answer sheet folded together with the answers out of view. The patient may check the answers when the crossword puzzle is completed.
4. Leave the "Controlling Hypertension" crossword puzzle with the patient.

By: Gaye Ragland, RN, BSN

CONTROLLING HYPERTENSION
Crossword Puzzle

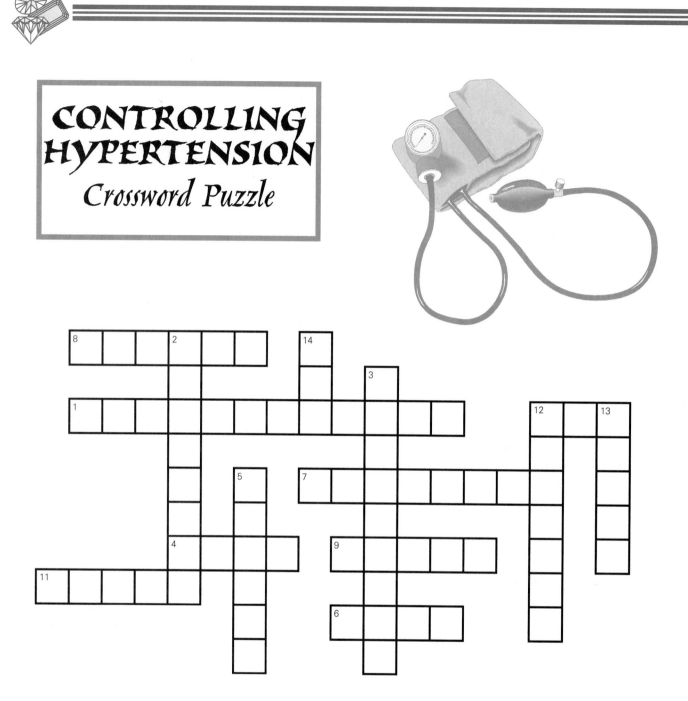

ACROSS

1. Another word for high blood pressure
4. The doctor often says cut this out
6. Causes of high blood pressure are called _____ factors
7. The top number
8. Try to reduce the _____ you are under
9. What you put on when you cheat on your diet.
11. Added stress may make your blood pressure problems _____
12. One of the risk factors having to do with your "birthday"

DOWN

2. Increase this only with your doctor's approval
3. The bottom number
5. Because there are often no symptoms of high blood pressure, it is called the _____ killer.
12. Heavy, regular drinking of this makes high blood pressure problems worse
13. Which adults should have their blood pressure checked
14. Who is at greater risk: men or women

212

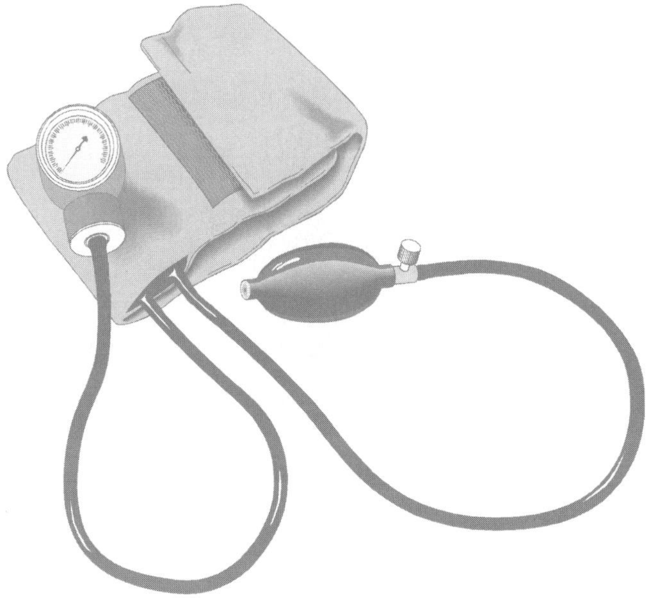

CONTROLLING HYPERTENSION

Crossword Puzzle

ANSWER KEY:

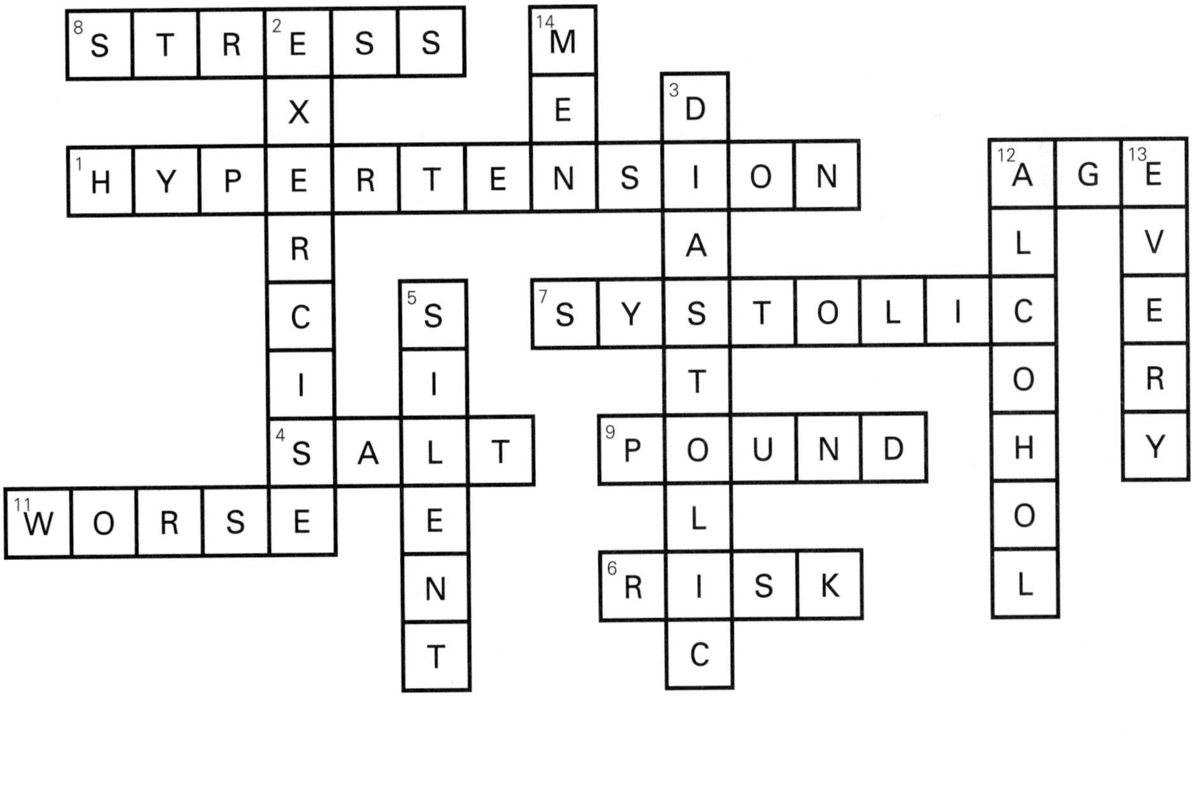

8 STRESS
14 MEN
3 DIASTOLIC
2 EXERCISE
1 HYPERTENSION
12 AGE
12 ALCOHOL
13 EVERY
5 SILENT
7 SYSTOLIC
4 SALT
9 POUND
11 WORSE
6 RISK

"RED HEART" COLLECTION

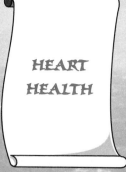

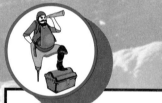

Treasure Chest

"'Red Heart' Collection"

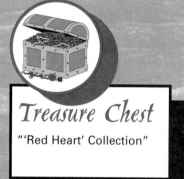

Educator Insights

As an icon use an empty box of red hots—instead of "red hots" call them "red hearts."

PREPARATION

1. Collect 6 to 8 visual aids that are red in color and shaped like a heart.
   Suggestions include but are not limited to:
   Red heart sticker
   Pencil with red hearts
   Red heart keychain
   Red heart lapel pin
   Red heart stationery
   Red heart sucker
   Red heart picture frame

IMPLEMENTATION

1. As you teach and reteach this treasure, have an ongoing collection of red heart icons.
2. Keep "Red Hearts" in a small box.
3. Precede the lesson by showing the patient your "red heart" collection.
4. Lead into "Heart Health" lesson by saying " . . . but these are not the red hearts I want to talk about. Today I want to talk about your 'Red Heart' . . ." You have your patient's attention and your heart health lesson is ready to begin.

By: Gaye Ragland, RN, BSN

CARDIAC CARTOON CAPERS

"The Story of Art"

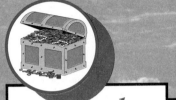

Treasure Chest

"Do You Know the Warning Signals Of A Heart Attack?"

"The Story of Art"

"The Story of Prudent Art"

Pen or pencil with an eraser

Educator Insights

Be sure to individualize the heart health teaching plan in accordance with the patient's specific doctor's orders.

PREPARATION

1. Copy and review "Do You Know the Warning Signals Of A Heart Attack?"
2. Copy and review "The Story of Art."
3. Copy and review "The Story of Prudent Art."
4. Make sure the patient has a pen or pencil with an eraser.

IMPLEMENTATION

1. Review "Do You Know Warning Signals Of A Heart Attack?" with the patient.
2. Review the "Story of Art" with the patient. Discuss the questions at the bottom of the page.
3. Review the "Story of Prudent Art" with the patient.
4. Discuss the questions at the bottom of the page.
5. Leave "Cardiac Cartoon Capers," "Cardiac Cartoon Capers" answer keys, and "Do You Know Warning Signals Of A Heart Attack?" with the patient.

By: Michelle Deck, MEd, BSN, RN, ACCE-R. Revised from "Cardiac Cartoon Capers." Instant Teaching Tools For Health Educators, *Mosby, St. Louis, 1995.*

Do You Know the Warning Signals of a

HEART ATTACK?

· ·

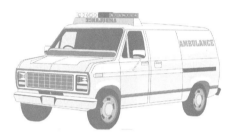

✓ Pressure in the chest.

✓ Discomfort in the chest.

✓ Fullness in the chest.

✓ Burning in the chest.

✓ Squeezing pain in the center of the chest.

✓ Pain in the center of the chest.

✓ Chest pain that radiates to the jaw and arm.

✓ Pain that spreads to the shoulders, neck, and arms.

✓ Chest discomfort that is associated with lightheadedness, fainting, sweating, nausea, or shortness of breath.

✓ Acute anxiety.

Not everyone will experience all of these symptoms listed above with every heart attack. If you are with someone experiencing the signs of a heart attack:

- Get help immediately
- Expect the patient to deny it is happening
- Call the emergency service or
- Get to the nearest 24 hour hospital that offers heart help
- Give cardiopulmonary resuscitation (CPR) if necessary

216

THE STORY OF ART

Art A. Tack is fifty-five years old. He smokes a pack of cigarettes a day and, as you can see, is a little overweight. Art is a "steak and potato" man and has felt no reason to change his diet up until now. His idea of exercise is getting up to find the TV remote control. At his recent check-up, his blood pressure was high (142/98) and his cholesterol was elevated above normal (310). He thought the numbers might mean something, so he played the lottery with them and won! But his luck is about to change. Unless he makes some lifestyle and dietary changes, Art is headed straight for a heart attack.

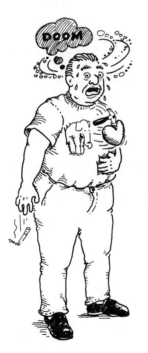

On the lines below, list some of the changes Art needs to make to become "heart healthy."

_____   _____

_____   _____

_____   _____

_____   _____

217

ANSWER SHEET 1:

The changes Art needs to make to become heart healthy:

1. **Stop smoking.** The cigarette smoking that Art is doing needs to be stopped. There is proof through research that smoking causes an increased risk of heart disease.

2. **Change his diet.** Art should reduce his intake of red meat (steak). Art should become diet conscious as he learns to reduce the cholesterol in his diet.

3. **Exercise with his doctor's permission.** Art should get more exercise than just operating the TV. As Art follows his doctor's instructions about exercise, he will increase his chances of getting his blood cholesterol under control.

4. **Control his high blood pressure.** Art should see his doctor for treatment of his high blood pressure. If Art is on medication for high blood pressure, he should have regular check-ups and take his prescribed medication exactly as it is ordered by his doctor.

5. Art must **realize that even winning the lottery will not produce the lifestyle changes that are necessary** for Art to have heart health. Lifestyle changes can only be made by Art.

THE STORY OF PRUDENT ART

Prudent Art is sixty-five years old. Ten years ago you saved his life when he had a heart attack. In gratitude, he split his lottery winnings with you. Since then, Art has been into prudent heart living. He is a slim, trim, active, nonsmoker. He has also started raising alligators as a pastime to decrease stress. He still occasionally has angina and takes nitroglycerine.

Today, he came home to find his favorite alligator, Fred, missing and a note that read:

> Dear Prudent Art,
>
> I have decided to move to Florida where the gators go wild.
> See you later, alligator.

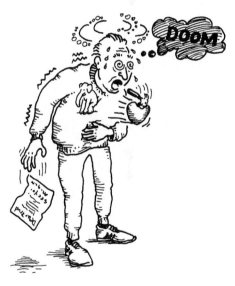

Prudent Art is distraught beyond limits. He is about to have his second heart attack. Here is a picture of him moments before his fateful second heart attack. See if you can identify the early warning signs.

You, thinking quickly, take the following actions:

1. _____

2. _____

3. _____

4. _____

219

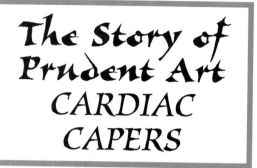

The Story of Prudent Art
CARDIAC CAPERS

The early warning signs of the heart attack about to hit Prudent Art:

1. Feeling of doom
2. Light-headedness (bubbles)
3. Dizziness (eyes twirling)
4. Jaw pain
5. Denial statement ("Don't worry. It's just indigestion.")
6. Sweating
7. Shoulder pain
8. Pounding heart (a hammer pounding)
9. Crushing chest pain (an elephant sitting on the chest)
10. Arm pain
11. Nausea

You, thinking quickly, take the following actions:

♦ Recognize what could be happening
♦ Reassure the patient and . . .
♦ Call for help (911 or your local emergency services number)
♦ Caregiver begin CPR, if needed

HEART ATTACK HIDEOUT

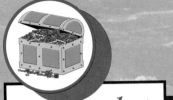

Treasure Chest

"Heart Attack Hideout"

"Heart Attack Hideout"
answer key

Pen or pencil with an
eraser

Educator Insights

To enhance learning, you
may choose to work the
puzzle with the patient
and discuss words as they
are located.

PREPARATION

1. Copy "Heart Attack Hideout" word search puzzle for the patient.
2. Copy the "Heart Attack Hideout" answer key.
3. Make sure the patient has a pen or pencil with an eraser.

IMPLEMENTATION

1. Ask the patient to complete the word search puzzle.
2. Explain that the hidden words are words associated with "Do You Know the Warning Signals of a Heart Attack?" on page 216.
3. Check the answer key with the patient when the word search is completed or leave the answer key folded together with the answers out of view. The patient may check the answers whenever the puzzle is completed.
4. Leave "Heart Attack Hideout" word search puzzle and answer key with the patient.

By: Gaye Ragland, RN, BSN

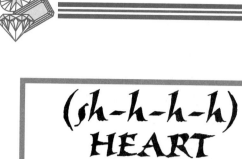

(sh-h-h-h) HEART ATTACK HIDEOUT Word Search

Directions: Using a colored marker, highlight each of the words associated with

"HEART ATTACK WARNINGS"

Remember: Words can be forward, backward, up and down, and diagonal.

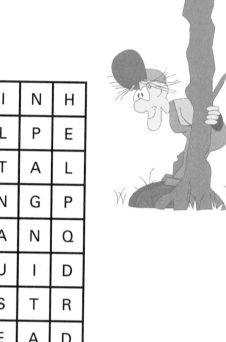

B	J	A	W	P	A	I	N	H
U	G	E	T	H	E	L	P	E
R	H	O	S	P	I	T	A	L
N	T	B	P	F	L	N	G	P
I	A	E	A	A	Q	A	N	Q
N	N	S	I	I	S	U	I	D
G	X	E	N	N	P	S	T	R
L	I	G	H	T	H	E	A	D
G	E	T	O	N	Z	A	E	E
S	T	R	E	S	S	T	W	N
B	Y	S	M	O	K	E	S	I
F	U	L	L	N	E	S	S	E
P	R	E	S	S	U	R	E	S

How many did you find? Are other **"Heart Attack Warning"** words hiding from you?

WORDS

Anxiety
Burning
Denies
Faint

Fullness
Get help
Hospital
Lighthead

Nausea
Obese
Pain
Pressure

Smokes
Stress
Sweating

222

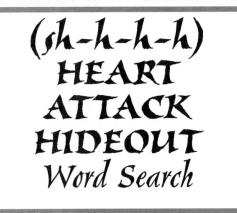

(sh-h-h-h)
HEART
ATTACK
HIDEOUT
Word Search

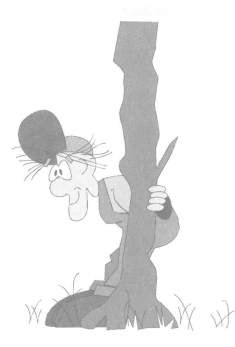

ANSWER KEY:

B	J	A	W	P	A	I	N	H
U	G	E	T	H	E	L	P	E
R	H	O	S	P	I	T	A	L
N	T	B	P	F	L	N	G	P
I	A	E	A	A	Q	A	N	Q
N	N	S	I	I	S	U	I	D
G	X	E	N	N	P	S	T	R
L	I	G	H	T	H	E	A	D
G	E	T	O	N	Z	A	E	E
S	T	R	E	S	S	T	W	N
B	Y	S	M	O	K	E	S	I
F	U	L	L	N	E	S	S	E
P	R	E	S	S	U	R	E	S

223

HEART JEOPARDY

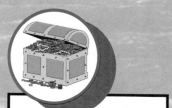

Treasure Chest

"Heart Jeopardy" quiz

"Heart Jeopardy" answer sheet

"Heart Jeopardy" award sheet

Red apple (optional)

Red paper (optional)

Pen or pencil with an eraser

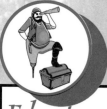

Educator Insights

Use red paper for red heart award sheet. Diet permitting, a red apple makes a nice reward.

PREPARATION

1. Copy and review "Heart Jeopardy" quiz.
2. Copy the "Heart Jeopardy" answer sheet.
3. Be sure the patient has a pen or pencil with an eraser.

IMPLEMENTATION

1. Ask the patient to complete the "Heart Jeopardy" quiz.
2. Explain that the patient will get 20 points for each correct answer.
3. Total the points as you check the answers.
4. Praise the patient for correct answers. Teach correct information for any missed answers.
5. Leave "Heart Jeopardy" and the reward sheet with the patient.

By: Gaye Ragland, RN, BSN

HEART JEOPARDY

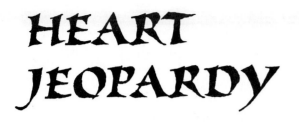

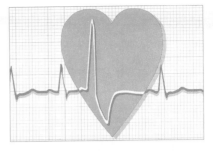

Directions: Answer the following questions. Check the answers when you are finished completing all the questions and total the points of those you get correct. ASK YOUR INSTRUCTOR ABOUT PRIZES.

20 points   1. If you are the child of either one or both parents with heart disease, the risk factor of _____ applies to you.

20 points   2. Do males or females have a greater risk of developing heart disease? _____

20 points   3. Do smokers have a higher or lower risk of developing heart disease? _____

20 points   4. People over the age of _____ have more heart attacks.

20 points   5. It is important that the level of blood _____ is kept within normal limits.

20 points   6. Name a way you reduce stress in your life: _____

20 points   7. Does stress have an effect on the risk for heart disease? _____

20 points   8. Are warning symptoms of high blood pressure always known? _____

20 points   9. Can all of the risk factors for developing heart disease be avoided? _____

20 points   10. Can some of the risk factors for developing heart disease be avoided? _____

20 points 11. Do blacks have a greater risk for developing heart disease? ♥

20 points 12. Too much alcohol can cause the blood pressure to rise and can eventually lead to heart ♥

20 points 13. If you have the disease ♥ (that affects your blood sugar), your risk of heart disease is greater.

20 points 14. What about physical activity with your doctor's approval? Is it good or bad for the heart? ♥

20 points 15. Cardiovascular (heart) disease is the number ♥ killer in the United States.

_____ **TOTAL POINTS**

226

HEART JEOPARDY

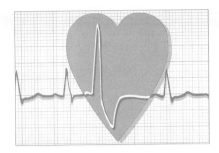

ANSWER SHEET:

20 points   1. If you are the child of either one or both parents with heart disease, the risk factor of **HEREDITY** applies to you.

20 points   2. Do males or females have a greater risk of developing heart disease? **MALES**

20 points   3. Do smokers have a higher or lower risk of developing heart disease? **HIGHER**

20 points   4. People over the age of **65** have more heart attacks.

20 points   5. It is important that the level of blood **CHOLESTEROL** is kept within normal limits.

20 points   6. Name a way you reduce stress in your life:

                _____

20 points   7. Does stress have an effect on the risk for heart disease? **YES**

20 points   8. Are warning symptoms of high blood pressure always known? **NO**

20 points   9. Can all of the risk factors for developing heart disease be avoided? **NO**

20 points   10. Can some of the risk factors for developing heart disease be avoided? **YES**

227

20 points 11. Do blacks have a greater risk for developing heart disease? **YES**

20 points 12. Too much alcohol can cause the blood pressure to rise and can eventually lead to heart **FAILURE**.

20 points 13. If you have the disease **DIABETES** (that affects your sugar), your risk of heart disease is greater.

20 points 14. What about physical activity with your doctor's approval? Is it good or bad for the heart? **GOOD**

20 points 15. Cardiovascular (heart) disease is the number **1** killer in the United States.

300 **TOTAL POINTS**

228

CONGRATULATIONS. YOU'RE A WINNER!

HEART JEOPARDY

0 to 100 points = heart-smart

100 to 200 points = heart-smarter

200 to 300 points = heart-smartest

MEET: HIATAL MABEL

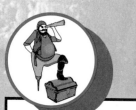

HIATAL
HERNIA

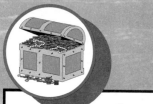

Treasure Chest

"How To Cradle That 'Hiatal' (hernia, that is)"

"Lifestyle and Dietary Behaviors" fact sheet

"Meet: Hiatal Mabel" question sheet

Pen or pencil with an eraser

Educator Insights

Assess the patient's eating habits. As you teach, target the areas which are critical to lifestyle management of the hiatal hernia.

PREPARATION

1. Copy and review "How To Cradle That 'Hiatal' (hernia, that is)".
2. Copy and review "Lifestyle and Dietary Behavior" fact sheet.
3. Copy and review "Meet: Hiatal Mabel" question sheet.
4. Make sure the patient has a pen or pencil with an eraser.

IMPLEMENTATION

1. Review "How To Cradle That 'Hiatal' (Hernia, that is)" with the patient.
2. Review "Lifestyle and Dietary Behaviors" fact sheet with the patient.
3. Give the patient "Meet: Hiatal Mabel" question sheet.
4. Ask the patient to complete the sheet by answering the questions verbally or in writing, or you may leave the sheet with the patient to be completed after the visit.
5. Leave "Meet: Hiatal Mabel," "How To Cradle That 'Hiatal,'" and "Lifestyle and Dietary Behaviors" with the patient.

By: Gaye Ragland, RN, BSN

How to Cradle that "Hiatal"

(Hernia, that is)

Just as an infant must be cradled for comfort, your hiatal hernia requires special care to keep symptoms to a minimum.

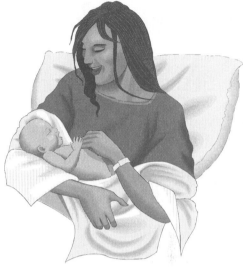

A "Hiatal Hernia" is a protrusion, or bulging of the stomach through the normal opening where the stomach joins the esophagus, or food pipe. Hiatal hernias are classified as either the rolling or the sliding type, but the majority are classified as sliding. Hiatal hernias are more likely to develop as you get older. Overweight people and women are more often affected.

Aging, injury, surgery, and curvature of the spine can contribute to the cause of a hiatal hernia. Whenever there is added pressure in the abdomen, the lower part of the food pipe and stomach may move upward into the chest. Some of the things that increase pressure inside the abdomen are coughing, bending, vomiting, pregnancy, severe exertion, wearing constricting clothing, straining, and extra weight.

Most people never even know they have a hiatal hernia. This is because most people are without symptoms of the hernia until they are bothered with heartburn or other symptoms associated with esophageal reflux. The presence of reflux symptoms often lead the doctor to suspect hiatal hernia. Esophageal reflux is the flowing back of the stomach contents into the esophagus (sometimes called the "food tube").

The sliding hiatal hernia moves upward into the chest when you lie down. When you stand or sit, the hernia moves downward again.

Some symptoms of reflux are heartburn, belching, regurgitation, hiccups, and even vomiting. It usually occurs 1 to 4 hours after eating and can be brought on by stress or by reclining after a meal.

The following page lists lifestyle and dietary changes that will help you manage your hiatal hernia as you try to keep symptoms to a minimum.

231

How to Cradle that "Hiatal"

(Hernia, that is)

LIFESTYLE AND DIETARY BEHAVIORS TO KEEP HIATAL HERNIA SYMPTOMS TO A MINIMUM

1. Follow the diet prescribed by your doctor.

2. Unless on another specified diet from your doctor, eat a high protein diet that is low in fat.

3. Eat small, frequent meals. Eat slowly and chew food well.

4. Limit foods that stimulate the production of gastric acid such as:

CHOCOLATE	FRUIT JUICES
ALCOHOL	NICOTINE
SPEARMINT	CAFFEINE
PEPPERMINT	SPICES

5. Drink water following the meal to rinse the esophagus or food pipe clean.

6. Do not lie down for 2 to 3 hours after eating.

7. Sleep on the right side. Elevate the head of the bed on blocks to prevent reflux at night. The worse the reflux, the higher the blocks, 4 to 10 inches.

8. Maintain weight within acceptable range.

9. Avoid bending, coughing, straining, lifting heavy objects, strenuous exercise, and wearing clothing that is too tight.

10. Take medications exactly as prescribed.

11. Do not eat fried or fatty foods.

12. Avoid any type of acidic foods.

232

MEET: HIATAL MABEL.

Directions: Please answer the following questions for Mabel as you share with her what you have learned about caring for your "hiatal" (hernia, that is!).

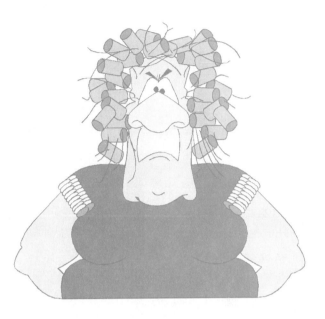

- My girdle helps me look **thinner.** Will it help my hiatal hernia, too?

- I love to eat fried chicken at the local "all you can eat" **fried** chicken bar. What about it?

- I heard that **chocolate** cures everything! Will it help my hiatal hernia?

- My doctor told me to **elevate** something in my house. Was it my refrigerator? How high?

- I like to sit right down, eat my meal and take a **nap** if I can. Is that good or bad?

- I've never been one to waste a lot of time at the table. I **eat** my meals **fast.** Is that how you do it?

- My doctor said to follow my meal with something. Since I can't remember what it was, will **coffee** work? What about **alcohol?**

- You say I should sleep on the **"right"** side. Now which side is the **right** one?

- To keep my breath fresh and clean, I eat **peppermint.** That will help . . . or will it hurt?

- Do I really need to **take the medicine** the doctor gave me, or will any old medicine do?

- My **weight is slightly more** than what it should be. Does that really matter?

233

WHAT ABOUT GOUT?

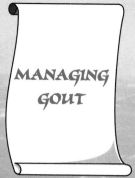

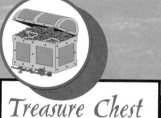

Treasure Chest

"What About Gout?"

"If You Have Gout."

"This Guy Has Gout."

Pen or pencil with an eraser

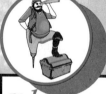

Educator Insights

Emphasize the importance of long term management of gout with the intent to prevent chronic complications.

PREPARATION

1. Review etiology, symptoms, treatment, and complications of gout.
2. Copy and review "What About Gout."
3. Copy and review "If You Have Gout."
4. Copy "This Guy Has Gout."
5. Make sure the patient has a pen or pencil with an eraser.

IMPLEMENTATION

1. Review "What About Gout?" with the patient.
2. Review "If You Have Gout" with the patient.
3. Review "This Guy Has Gout" with the patient.
4. Suggest posting "If You Have Gout" in the kitchen (e.g., on the refrigerator door).
5. Leave "This Guy Has Gout" with the patient to serve as a follow up lesson on gout information.

By: Gaye Ragland, RN, BSN

WHAT ABOUT GOUT?

"Gout" is a form of arthritis that affects 1.6 million people in the United States. It affects mostly men (90%) and usually the persons affected are over thirty years of age. In past history gout has been considered to be a disease of kings and queens, since the disease was associated with the eating of a high protein diet afforded only by the rich.

Either foods with too much purine in the diet or the body's inability to break down the purine results in the formation of uric acid crystals. These crystals lodge in the joints and connective tissue. The most common joint affected is in the great toe. Other joints may be affected, like the knees, wrists, and ankles.

Acute attacks commonly begin at night, but may occur at any time and at irregular intervals. They usually last from three to seven days. Acute episodes occur suddenly with a severely painful joint that is red, warm, tender, and has limited movement. There are a number of factors that can bring on an attack, including a high intake of purines, excessive alcohol consumption, stress, or severe illness.

Treatment for gout includes diet, medications, and resting the sore joint. Dietary treatment is aimed at weight reduction, if necessary, limitation of alcohol, and limited purine intake. It is important to drink enough fluids. Ask your doctor or nurse if you need to limit your food or fluid intake for other reasons. Fluids help prevent kidney stones from developing. Medications can be prescribed to reduce inflammation and prevent future attacks in patients who have multiple yearly attacks.

Treatment for an acute attack of gout includes bedrest. It is important to keep the affected joint elevated. It may be necessary to use a bed cradle to prevent the bed linens from touching the painful joint. Remember, continuing to bear weight causes increased pain as well as further deterioration of the joint.

It is important that gout be controlled. Uncontrolled gout can lead to an ongoing, chronic disease that is not only painful but causes severe joint deformity and loss of function. It is important to follow the plan of treatment your doctor has prescribed for you.

Copyright © 1996 by Mosby–Year Book, Inc.

If you have gout. . .

✓ whole milk

✓ poultry

✓ bacon, bacon fat, fat back, salt pork

✓ bouillon, meat drippings, meat gravies

✓ all breads made with yeast

✓ wild game

✓ liver, kidney, heart, brain, sweetbreads

✓ anchovies, sardines, fish roe, shrimp, herring, mackerel

✓ dried beans and peas

✓ asparagus, mushrooms, spinach

. . . Leave these foods out!!!

THIS GUY HAS GOUT.

- ◆ How old are people who usually have gout?

- ◆ Gout is a form of what illness?

- ◆ Why was gout considered a disease of the rich?

- ◆ What areas of the body are most affected?

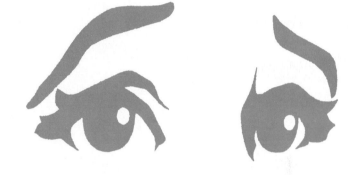

- ◆ Which joint is most commonly affected?

- ◆ What things could have brought on this guy's attack?

- ◆ What kind of diet should he follow?

- ◆ What is the treatment that his doctor would probably prescribe?

- ◆ Why should he follow the doctor's orders?

STRIKE OUT GOUT

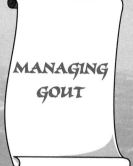
PREPARATION

1. Copy "Strike Out Gout" word search puzzle.
2. Copy the "Strike Out Gout" answer key.
3. Make sure the caregiver has a pen or pencil with an eraser.

IMPLEMENTATION

1. Ask the patient to complete the word search puzzle.
2. Explain that the words hidden are the names of foods to be left out if you have gout.
3. Check the answers when the patient finishes the puzzle or leave the answer sheet folded together with the answers out of view. The patient may check the answers whenever the puzzle is completed.

By: Gaye Ragland, RN, BSN

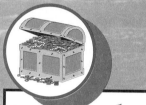

Treasure Chest

"Strike Out Gout" word search puzzle

"Strike Out Gout" answer key

Pen or pencil with an eraser

Educator Insights

Have the patient identify which, if any, of the foods named in the puzzle are foods the patient eats frequently.

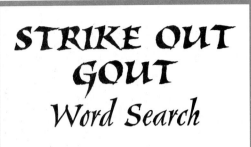

STRIKE OUT GOUT
Word Search

Directions: Strike a line through each of the names of foods to be "left out" if you have "gout."

Remember: The words may be spelled forward, backward, up and down, and diagonal.

W	O	H	I	Y	E	N	D	I	K
A	H	P	G	A	M	E	N	S	Y
S	P	O	R	K	P	N	Y	F	E
P	Z	U	L	Q	P	P	V	A	A
A	Q	L	N	E	Q	O	A	T	S
R	L	T	I	S	M	L	R	B	T
A	M	R	A	T	Z	I	G	A	B
G	N	Y	R	E	V	I	L	C	R
U	O	C	B	A	C	O	N	K	E
S	A	R	D	I	N	E	S	O	A
A	D	B	S	H	R	I	M	P	D
D	R	I	E	D	P	E	A	S	T

WORDS

Asparagus
Bacon
Brain
Dried Peas

Fat Back
Game
Gravy
Kidney

Liver
Pork
Poultry
Sardines

Shrimp
Whole Milk
Yeast Bread

239

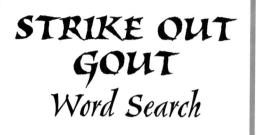

STRIKE OUT GOUT
Word Search

ANSWER KEY:

W	O	H	I	Y	E	N	D	I	K
A	H	P	G	A	M	E	N	S	Y
S	P	O	R	K	P	N	Y	F	E
P	Z	U	L	Q	P	P	V	A	A
A	Q	L	N	E	Q	O	A	T	S
R	L	T	I	S	M	L	R	B	T
A	M	R	A	T	Z	I	G	A	B
G	N	Y	R	E	V	I	L	C	R
U	O	C	B	A	C	O	N	K	E
S	A	R	D	I	N	E	S	O	A
A	D	B	S	H	R	I	M	P	D
D	R	I	E	D	P	E	A	S	T

240

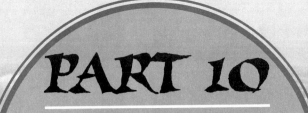

PART 10

Instant Treasures for Everything Else

SOAKING IT UP

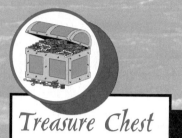

Treasure Chest

2 sponges about
4 inches × 6 inches

Marker

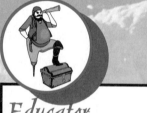

Educator Insights

Be sure to use a laundry-type marker that will not wash off the sponge. You may wish to give the patient the sponge to keep as a reminder of high-sodium foods that are to be avoided. If so, be sure to list the particular patient's greatest "salty temptations."

PREPARATION

1. Obtain 2 sponges (car-washing type), preferably in different colors.
2. On the front of one of the sponges print a listing of commonly eaten high-sodium foods. Let it dry completely before using it.

IMPLEMENTATION

1. As you teach the principle of fluid retention, produce the two sponges and allow the patient to hold them.
2. Relate the retention of fluid in the tissue to the retention of water in a sponge.
3. Move with the patient to the nearest sink. Ask the patient to wet the sponge that has the listing of high sodium foods.
4. Ask the patient to compare the weights of the wet and dry sponges. As the patient equates the heavier sponge to the one retaining the water, explain the extra workload on the body systems when body tissues weigh more due to an accumulation of excess fluid.

By: Gaye Ragland, RN, BSN

SPRING HAS SPRUNG

PREPARATION

1. Obtain one Slinky® toy (a long, expandable plastic coil-type toy).

IMPLEMENTATION

1. As you teach peristalsis of the intestines, demonstrate the relaxing and contraction movement by stretching the Slinky® toy.
2. Let the patient hold the Slinky® and stretch and contract the toy as you talk about the "spring" in the intestines.

By: Gaye Ragland, RN, BSN

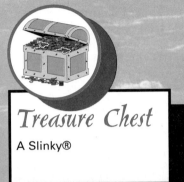

Treasure Chest

A Slinky®

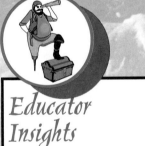

Educator Insights

This also works well as you teach skin turgor.

BIG RED

PREPARATION

1. Obtain one large pair of red nylon underwear (e.g., queen size 3X). Check a local dollar store for a pair under $5.00.

IMPLEMENTATION

1. As you begin teaching constipation, have large red underwear hidden out of sight.
2. Talk about the loss of elasticity in the normally stretchy intestine that stretches and relaxes to move the feces along the way toward elimination. Emphasize the phrase "loss of elasticity."
3. As you present the large red underwear, relate the loss of elasticity to the loss of elastic in underwear after they become old and worn out.
4. Continue the lesson by explaining that the result of this loss of elasticity is slower-moving feces through the intestines. Explain that the extra time the feces remains in the intestines allows more time for the water in the stool to be absorbed, resulting in a hard, dry stool.
5. If inadequate fluid intake is a problem, use this activity to stress how the water is absorbed from the stool because of the sluggishness of the intestines (due to the loss of elasticity).
6. Give specific instructions, in accordance with specific diet orders, for increasing fluids.

By: Gaye Ragland, RN, BSN

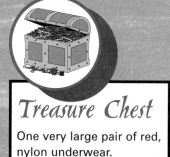

Treasure Chest

One very large pair of red, nylon underwear.

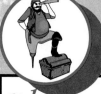

Educator Insights

Use this teaching icon on selected patients. Be ready to laugh!

244

THE PROCESS OF ELIMINATION

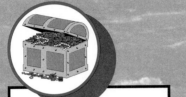

Treasure Chest

"Moving Right Along"

"The Process of Elimination"

"The Process of Elimination" answer key

Pen or pencil with an eraser

Educator Insights

Use large, red underwear (see "Big Red" page 244) or Slinky® for teaching icon, if desired.

PREPARATION

1. Copy and review "Moving Right Along."
2. Copy and review "The Process of Elimination."
3. Copy "The Process of Elimination" answer key.
4. Make sure the patient has a pen or pencil with an eraser.

IMPLEMENTATION

1. Discuss "Moving Right Along" with the patient as you teach constipation.
2. When finished, ask the patient to complete "The Process of Elimination." Assist the patient if necessary.
3. Leave "Moving Right Along" and "The Process of Elimination" with the patient.

By: Gaye Ragland, RN, BSN

Moving Right Along

COPING WITH CONSTIPATION

Constipation occurs when the feces (semi-solid waste that is eliminated by your body) moves slowly through the intestinal tract. This slow movement allows the water in the feces to be absorbed, and causes the feces to become dried and hard and results in constipation.

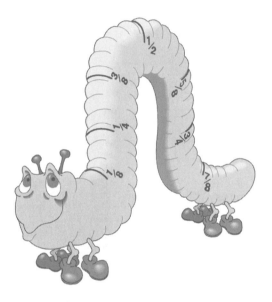

Feces is moved through the intestines by peristalsis (or smooth muscle contractions). As your intestines relax and contract in an "inchworm" type of movement, the feces is pushed along until it finally reaches the rectum where it is stored until it is time to be eliminated from the body. When elimination takes place, this is called a "bowel movement" and the eliminated feces is called "stool."

Some causes of constipation are too little bulk in the diet, not drinking enough liquids, not eating enough food, taking certain medications, frequent use of laxatives, and holding back a bowel movement when the urge strikes. Constipation can also be caused by age. As a person grows older, the intestines lose some of their elasticity (the ability to stretch). This natural loss of elasticity slows down the movement of the feces through the intestines and can cause hard dried stools. This can make bowel movements difficult and sometimes painful.

Constipation means different things to different people. Some people feel that they should have a bowel movement every day, and anything less is cause for concern. Some people have more than one bowel movement a day. And still others have a bowel movement only every two or three days. Some people have bowel movements at night and others have bowel movements in the morning. This routine of bowel elimination differs from person to person.

Many older people expect constipation to be a problem that will come naturally as they age. However, all older people do not have problems with constipation. Ask your doctor or nurse if you feel you need a laxative or stool softener to help with constipation problems.

When considering bowel function, the frequency of bowel movements, the color, the consistency (liquid or hard), the odor, and the amount should all be considered. And all of these aspects of bowel function can be affected by many factors, both psychological and physical.

A well-balanced diet plays an important role in normal bowel function. Foods that are high in fiber tend to hold water in the stool. This makes the stool softer and easier to pass. If you are able to chew and swallow adequately and your diet permits, consider the following foods that may be added to your diet to promote good bowel elimination: **slow-cooked oatmeal, whole-grain cereals, prunes, carrots, cabbage,** and **unpeeled fruits and vegetables**. Be sure to drink enough fluids.

Activity, when approved by your doctor, helps you to maintain muscle tone and stimulates the peristalsis or smooth muscle activity that keeps the feces moving through the intestines. Walking, and even approved exercises for the bed patient, may be of benefit to keep the bowels moving.

Even though the function of your bowels is a very private matter, it is most important to discuss with your doctor any problems or concerns about your elimination. Remember, the ability for your body to remove waste is very important to your well-being.

THE PROCESS OF ELIMINATION

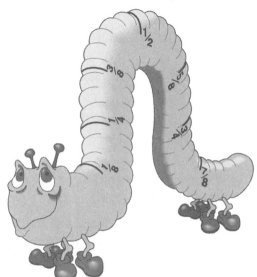

Instructions: Match the following phrases on the left with the correct word on the right.

_____ 1. The symptom of this disorder is a hard, dry stool.

A. Well-balanced

_____ 2. What feces is called once it leaves the body.

B. Elasticity

_____ 3. The "inchworm" type movement that pushes feces through the intestines.

C. Exercise

_____ 4. What there is less of in the intestines when a person becomes older.

D. Stool

_____ 5. The word meaning whether the stool is hard or liquid.

E. Peristalsis

_____ 6. The best type of diet to aid in the process of elimination.

F. Rectum

_____ 7. Foods that are high in this cannot be digested completely.

G. Consistency

_____ 8. Where feces is stored until it is time for the feces to be eliminated from the body.

H. Doctor or nurse

_____ 9. What helps maintain muscle tone and should only be done if it is approved by your doctor.

I. Constipation

_____10. Who to ask if you have problems with elimination.

J. Fiber

248

THE PROCESS OF ELIMINATION

ANSWER KEY

I 1. The symptom of this disorder is a hard, dry stool.

A. Well-balanced

D 2. What feces is called once it leaves the body.

B. Elasticity

E 3. The "inchworm" type movement that pushes feces through the intestines.

C. Exercise

B 4. What there is less of in the intestines when a person becomes older.

D. Stool

G 5. The word meaning whether the stool is hard or liquid.

E. Peristalsis

A 6. The best type of diet to aid in the process of elimination.

F. Rectum

J 7. Foods that are high in this cannot be digested completely.

G. Consistency

F 8. Where feces is stored until time it is for the feces to be eliminated from the body.

H. Doctor or nurse

C 9. What helps maintain muscle tone and should only be done if it is approved by your doctor.

I. Constipation

H 10. Who to ask if you have problems with elimination.

J. Fiber

249

WHAT'S UP DOC?

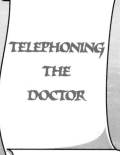

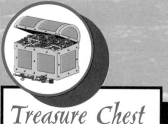

Treasure Chest

"What's Up Doc?" fact sheet

"What's Up Doc?" telephone checklist

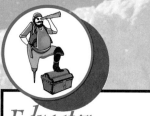

Educator Insights

If your employer gives away complimentary pens, pencils, or notepads, consider giving these items to the patient as you teach this treasure.

PREPARATION

1. Copy and review "What's Up Doc?" fact sheet.
2. Copy "What's Up Doc?" telephone checklist.
3. Make 10 duplicate copies to leave in the patient's home.

IMPLEMENTATION

1. Discuss "What's Up Doc?" with the patient and/or caregiver.
2. Go over "What's Up Doc?" telephone checklist with the patient and the caregiver.
3. Leave "What's Up Doc?" in the patient's home. Include 10 copies of the telephone checklist placed in a folder.
4. Ask the patient and/or caregiver to identify a safe location near the telephone for the spare checklists.

By: Susan Lofton, MSN, RN

WHAT'S UP DOC?

A Practical Guide for Use When Telephoning Your Doctor . . .

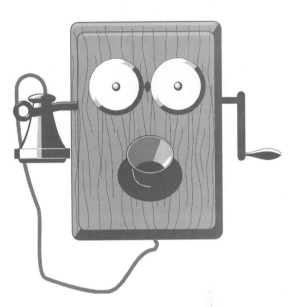

BEFORE THE CALL:

- Organize your thoughts! Take a moment to decide just what facts you need to tell your doctor and exactly what questions you must ask your doctor.
- Write down any questions that you want answered.
- Keep your pencil and pad of paper beside the phone to record information your doctor will give you in return.
- Make a list of all your current medicines. Don't forget to include any over-the-counter medications that you regularly take.
- Your doctor will need the name of your pharmacy. Have the name and phone number of your pharmacy in front of you before you call the doctor.

DURING THE CALL:

- If the call is of an urgent nature, tell the receptionist who answers the phone. Be specific on the nature of your call. If you are experiencing any sudden pain(s) or new symptoms, tell the nurse that you need to speak with your doctor immediately.
- Give the nurse a reliable phone number where the doctor can return your call. Remain at that number until your call is returned. Keep the phone line clear until the doctor is able to return your call.
- Speak clearly and distinctly to your doctor. State your symptoms, answer the doctor's questions, and ask those questions which you have already written down. Respect your doctor's time by remaining on the subject. This is not a social call.
- Before ending the call, take another moment to consider the information and instructions the doctor gave you. This is the time to get clear instructions on any information that you do not understand. Repeat back to the doctor any instructions given to you.

251

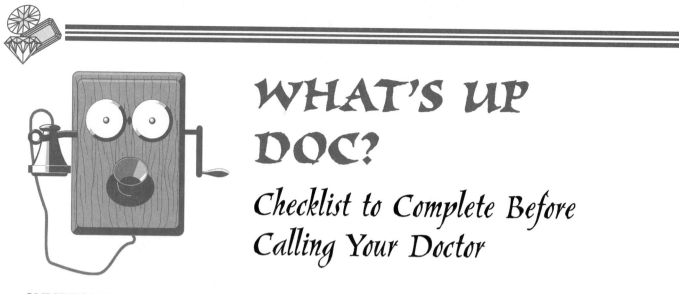

WHAT'S UP DOC?

Checklist to Complete Before Calling Your Doctor

SYMPTOMS: (Include temperature, unusual or sudden pain, site of discomfort, how long you have been experiencing this problem):

_____

_____

LIST OF CURRENT MEDICATIONS:

Medicine: Dosage:

_____

_____

_____

Allergies: _____

LOCAL PHARMACY AND PHONE NUMBER: _____

NUMBER WHERE YOU CAN BE REACHED BY YOUR DOCTOR: _____

QUESTIONS FOR YOUR DOCTOR:

_____

_____

_____

252

THE CANDIED TRUTH ABOUT CANES

PREPARATION

1. Copy and review "The Candied Truth About Canes."
2. Obtain an additional assistive device, if possible (other than the patient's personal one).

IMPLEMENTATION

1. Review "The Candied Truth About Canes" with the patient.
2. Demonstrate ambulation for the patient, using correct ambulation techniques.
3. Have the patient, if able, return the demonstration.
4. Remember, demonstrate exactly. The patient will copy what he sees.
5. Leave "The Candied Truth About Canes" with the patient.

By: Gaye Ragland, RN, BSN

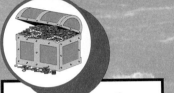

Treasure Chest

"The Candied Truth About Canes"

Assistive device specifically ordered for the patient

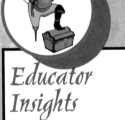

Educator Insights

It is usually not too difficult to find a cane or a walker tucked away in a storage room or supply closet. The patient can better mimic you if each of you use one for the lesson.

THE CANDIED TRUTH ABOUT CANES (AND WALKERS)

Your cane or walker (circle one) is a piece of equipment that your doctor ordered for you to help support you as you walk.

Cane: Use your cane on your stronger side. Keep the tip(s) of the cane about 6–10 inches to the side of the body and about 6 inches in front of the foot. This will help you balance your weight between the cane and your weak side. As you start to walk, move the cane forward about 12 inches. Next, bring the weak foot forward to the cane. Now place the stronger foot in front of both the cane and the weak foot.

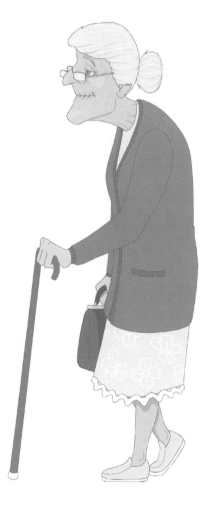

Walker: Your walker was ordered to help with your balance or to support your weight as you walk or both. Most people feel more secure with the walker than with other devices. The walker is picked up and moved about 6 inches at a time. As you walk toward it, hold onto it securely. Do not push down on your walker for support unless all four legs of the walker are resting evenly on the ground. When you are moving the walker, your feet must be planted firmly on the ground and you should be standing still. When you move your feet, your walker must be planted firmly on level ground and all four legs should be resting on even ground. Do not slide or drag the walker along the ground. Wear sturdy, non-skid shoes.

It is important that your assistive device is adjusted for your height. The hand piece should be level with your hip so that when you hold onto it you have a slight bend in your elbow.

Whether you use a cane or a walker, remember, the device is not to help you stand up from a sitting position. It is to help support you while you walk.

254

PILLOW TALK

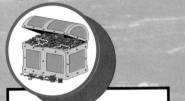

Treasure Chest

"Pillow Talk: How To Get A Good Night's Sleep"

"Pillow Talk: How I Will Get A Good Night's Sleep"

Pen or pencil with an eraser

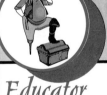

Educator Insights

Mention to the patient how refreshing it is to sleep on clean sheets (line-dried ones are especially nice!)

PREPARATION

1. Copy and review "Pillow Talk: How To Get A Good Night's Sleep."
2. Copy and review "Pillow Talk: How I Will Get A Good Night's Sleep."
3. Make sure the patient has a pen or pencil with an eraser.

IMPLEMENTATION

1. Discuss "Pillow Talk: How To Get A Good Night's Sleep" with the patient.
2. Discuss the patient's particular sleeping problems. Assess the patient's sleep environment and offer suggestions that may promote better rest.
3. Have the patient complete "Pillow Talk: How I Will Get A Good Night's Sleep."
4. Leave "Pillow Talk: How To Get a Good Night's Sleep" and "Pillow Talk: How I Will Get A Good Night's Sleep" with the patient.

By: Gaye Ragland, RN, BSN

PILLOW TALK

HOW TO GET A GOOD NIGHT'S SLEEP

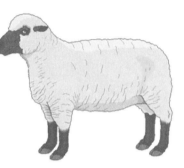

1. Establish a routine for bedtime, including a routine time to retire.

2. If possible, do not use the bedroom for anything except sleeping.

3. Wear comfortable night clothing. Some people prefer nylon or satin fabric. Other people prefer cotton or flannel. Consider your body temperature comfort zone as you make your choice.

4. Set your thermostat to maintain a temperature suited to your comfort a few minutes before retiring.

5. Eliminate caffeine from the afternoon and throughout the evening. Remember, caffeinated coffee is not the only source of caffeine. Restrict caffeinated tea and chocolate as well. Check with your pharmacist about over-the-counter medications that contain caffeine.

6. Take a warm bath at bedtime.

7. Have your caregiver give you a backrub.

8. Soft music at bedtime may help you relax.

9. Try drinking a glass of warm milk or other warm beverage (diet permitting).

10. Eat a light snack (diet permitting). Milk products, cheese and beef are especially good.

11. Do deep breathing exercises by taking in a deep breath and blowing it out slowly as you let your muscles relax.

12. Try using imagery. Imagine positive thoughts like a favorite vacation spot or a very pleasant past event. By filling your mind with pleasant thoughts, you will leave no room for unpleasant thoughts to sneak into your mind.

13. If the face of your clock glows in the dark, turn the clock out of sight or cover it up. Position so that you cannot see it if you awaken during the night.

14. Limit the amount of time you nap during the day. Though napping is useful, your nap should not last longer than two hours.

15. If you retire for the night a little later than usual, get up about the same time as usual. Once you wake up, go ahead and get out of bed. If you wake up during the night and are unable to go back to sleep, get up after 30 minutes. Read or find a quiet activity that you can do in another room of the house.

16. Remember, alcohol may result in early waking and nicotine is a stimulant.

17. If your bedtime must change, try to continue rising at the same time, maintaining a routine sleep/wake cycle.

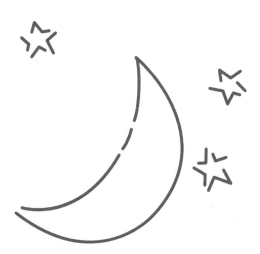

. . . . PLEASANT DREAMS

PILLOW TALK

HOW I WILL GET A GOOD NIGHT'S SLEEP:

1. I will nap for only _____ hours a day.

2. I will wear _____ for sleep clothes.

3. I will set the thermostat at _____.

4. I will eliminate caffeine after _____ o'clock in the afternoon.

5. I will cover the face of the clock if it glows in the dark.

6. I will do the following before I go to bed:
   (check the ones that apply)

   Take a warm bath.

   Have a backrub.

   Listen to soft music.

   Drink a glass of _____ _____.

   Eat a snack.

   Do deep breathing exercises.

   Use imagery to relax.

7. I will go to bed at _____ p.m.

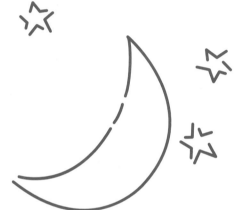

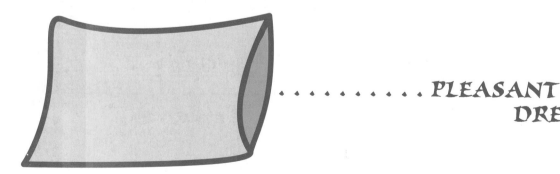

. . . . *PLEASANT DREAMS*

258

BOTTLED BLUES

Treasure Chest

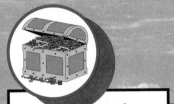

Small strips of blue paper

Large pill bottle or baby food jar

Pen or pencil with an eraser

Marker pen

Educator Insights

Be a good listener throughout the exercise. The patient may cry or even express anger. Listen attentively and be supportive. Keep the dialogue open.

PREPARATION

1. Cut five to ten strips of blue paper.
2. Obtain a large pill bottle or baby food jar.
3. Label the jar with a piece of paper or gauze tape with the words "BOTTLED BLUES."
4. Make sure the patient has a pen or pencil with an eraser.

IMPLEMENTATION

1. Initiate discussion with the patient about the most difficult aspects of chronic illness.
2. Ask the patient to write those things that cause him to worry and feel blue on the strips of blue paper. Assist the patient, if necessary.
3. After the patient writes the "worries" on 4 or 5 of the blue paper strips of paper, put the worry strips into the "Bottled Blues" bottle.
4. Bring to the patient's attention those "worries" which the patient cannot control.
5. Talk about stress relieving techniques.
6. When the discussion is complete have the patient discard the "Bottled Blues" in the trash.
7. Conclude with relaxing, deep-breathing exercises.

By: Susan Lofton, RN, MSN

A "HAIR RAISING" EXPERIENCE

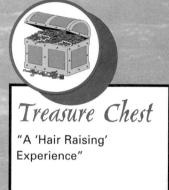

Treasure Chest

"A 'Hair Raising' Experience"

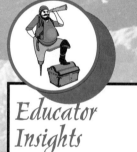

Educator Insights

Be alert to signs of distress about present or anticipated hair loss. Encourage the patient to express fear and seek answers to questions.

PREPARATION

1. Copy and review "A 'Hair Raising' Experience."

IMPLEMENTATION

1. Review "A 'Hair Raising' Experience" with the patient.
2. Seek answers to any questions the patient has about hair loss, present or anticipated.
3. Listen attentively for cues of distress about hair loss. Be supportive.
4. Seek information about hair loss from the American Cancer Society.
5. Leave "A 'Hair Raising' Experience" with the patient.

By: Gaye Ragland, RN, BSN

A "HAIR RAISING" EXPERIENCE

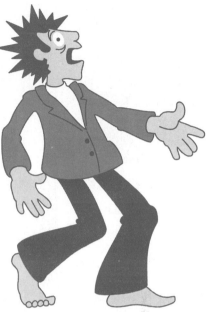

Hair loss can occur from certain drugs, disease, and has even been linked to stress. When some people learn they have cancer, the fear of hair loss as a side effect of chemotherapy is one of the early concerns that comes to mind. Because the hair has such a profound influence on the facial image as well as the entire image of the body, the uncertainty of the look without hair can be frightening.

Aside from the misgivings of the changed appearance, another aspect of hair loss is that of discomfort. The loss of hair can cause the head to be left cold and can even result in a sunburn of the scalp. If you have a condition that affects hair growth or causes possible loss of your hair, the following facts will hopefully make dealing with hair loss a little less unpleasant.

- Share any concerns or fears about hair loss with your doctor.
- Take with you to the doctor a written list of questions about your condition and any questions about your hair that may be of concern to you.
    "How soon will my hair begin to come out?"
    "Will my hair grow back?"
    "How soon will my hair grow back?"
    "When my hair grows back, will it look the same?"
    "Should I expect to lose my body hair?"
    "Will my hair all come out at one time, or should I expect it to come out gradually?"
- Use a mild shampoo and conditioner. This will keep the hair cells nourished.
- Do not use hair barrettes, hair dryers, curling irons, electric rollers, hair bands, or rubber bands in the hair.
- Avoid using hair dyes, permanent waves, or hair sprays.
- Sleep on a satin pillowcase to prevent rubbing of the hair against the linens during sleeping.
- Use a wide-toothed comb or a soft-bristled brush for hair care.
- Buy a wig, scarf, or cap before the hair starts to fall out.
- If you plan to buy a wig, do so before your hair falls out. You will be able to better match both color and texture.
- Cover the head with a light scarf or hat if out in the sun.
- Cover the head with a hat or cap if out in the cold.

THIS IS A
RECORDING

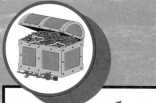

Treasure Chest

"This Is A Recording"

Pen or pencil with an eraser

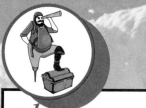

Educator Insights

Remind the patient to keep the record in a private place, if desired. Also, remind the patient/caregiver to record questions and comments as they occur.

PREPARATION

1. Copy pages 1 and 2 of "This Is A Recording."
2. Make sure the patient/caregiver has a pen or pencil with an eraser for recording information onto the record form.

IMPLEMENTATION

1. Explain to the patient/caregiver the importance of recording useful medical information.
2. Instruct the patient/caregiver to record information in a timely manner so it is not forgotten.
3. Instruct the patient/caregiver to show the record to the nurse and to carry the record when visiting the doctor or going to the hospital.

By: Gaye Ragland, RN, BSN

THIS IS A RECORDING . . . OF MY MEDICAL HAPPENINGS FOR THE MONTH OF _____

MY NAME _____

PHYSICIAN _____**; DATE OF NEXT MD. VISIT** _____

CURRENT MEDICATIONS:

_____

_____

_____

_____

_____

_____

CHANGES IN MY ROUTINE PRESCRIPTIONS THIS MONTH:

_____

_____

_____

_____

OVER-THE-COUNTER MEDICINE I HAVE TAKEN THIS MONTH:

_____

_____

_____

PROBLEMS WITH URINATION:

_____

PROBLEMS WITH BOWEL MOVEMENTS:

_____

FREQUENCY OF BOWEL MOVEMENTS: _____

_____

PROBLEMS WITH SLEEPING:

_____

PROBLEMS WITH EATING:

_____

SORES OR WOUNDS THAT WILL NOT HEAL:

_____

PROBLEMS WITH NERVOUSNESS OR DEPRESSION:

_____

FAMILY PROBLEMS THAT I FEEL ARE AFFECTING MY HEALTH:

_____

_____

NEW PROBLEMS I WANT TO DISCUSS:

_____

_____

_____

_____

QUESTIONS I HAVE ABOUT MY ILLNESS OR MY MEDICATIONS:

_____

_____

_____

_____

ELIMINATION RECORD

Directions: Mark each time the patient urinates. Describe bowel movements as large or small, soft, hard, or liquid. Make notes of anything unusual.

Date	Urinates	Bowel Movement
SUN		
MON		
TUE		
WED		
THU		
FRI		
SAT		
SUN		
MON		
TUE		
WED		
THU		
FRI		
SAT		

265

SCAVENGER HUNT BREAST EXAM

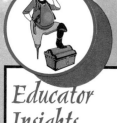

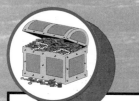

Treasure Chest

"Self-Examination of the Breasts"

"The BESt Time for BSE"

"Scavenger Hunt Breast Exam"

"Scavenger Hunt Breast Exam" answer key

Red marking pen

Educator Insights

A review of this procedure can be found in almost all medical-surgical texts. Additional BSE material can also be obtained from the American Cancer Society.

PREPARATION

1. Review and copy "Self-Examination of the Breasts."
2. Review and copy "The BESt Time for BSE."
3. Review and copy "Scavenger Hunt Breast Exam."
4. Copy the "Scavenger Hunt Breast Exam" answer key.
5. Make sure the patient has a red marking pen.

IMPLEMENTATION

1. Teach patient breast self-examination techniques using "Self-Examination of the Breasts" teaching treasure.
2. Teach the patient recommendations for breast exam frequency and tips for remembering a monthly examine routine using "The BESt Time for BSE" treasure.
3. Instruct the patient to complete the "Scavenger Hunt Breast Exam," assisting the patient if necessary.
4. Make sure the following **important** points are taught and understood:
   - Breast exam in each of the various positions as outlined in the "Self-Examination of the Breasts" treasure
   - What to look for
   - Changes and/or abnormal findings reported to a physician
   - Guidelines for a mammogram
5. Leave "Self Examination of the Breasts," "The BESt Time For BSE," "Scavenger Hunt Breast Exam," and "Scavenger Hunt Breast Exam," answer key with the patient.

By: Gaye Ragland, RN, BSN

Self-Examination of the Breasts

WHEN TO EXAMINE
- Examine the breasts at least monthly.
- The best time to examine the breasts is monthly when the breasts are not swollen or tender, usually 7 to 10 days after your period.
- If your periods are not regular or if you no longer have a period, be sure to examine your breasts on the same day each month.

HOW TO EXAMINE
In front of a mirror:
- Examine the breasts with the arms hanging loosely at the sides.
- Examine the breasts with the arms stretched out over the head.
- Examine the breasts with the hands pressed together in front of the chest.
- Examine the breasts while sitting down.
- Examine the breasts while leaning forward.

Lying down:
- In this position, place a pillow under your right shoulder, put your right arm behind your head and use your left hand to examine the right breast. When the examination of the right breast is completed, place the pillow under your left shoulder, put your left arm behind your head and use your right hand to examine the left breast.

WHAT TO LOOK FOR
- Look at the size of the breasts. Is one breast unusually larger than the other. Does anything look different from the month before?
- Do the breasts look alike?
- Is there puckering or dimpling?
- Are there any spots that are discolored or any spots where the color has changed?
- As you look at the nipples and the dark area around the nipples, do you notice any change?
- Examine these areas for similarity, color, texture, size, nipples turned inward, or nipples pointing in a different direction than usual.
- Feel for lumps or thickening in the breasts. The more you practice Breast Self Exam, the more accustomed you will become to the way your breasts feel. You will be more likely to notice a change in your breast from one month to the next.

HOW TO EXAMINE

1. Have your instructor identify the boundaries that are to be examined. Boundaries include the areas under the arms to the mid-sternum (chest), and the area above and within the collarbone. (See boundary area of drawing on page 271.) Check these areas for enlarged lymph nodes, masses, or tenderness.
2. Feel your breast using the pads of your fingers. (The pad of the finger is the top one-third of the finger.) Ask your instructor to show you how much pressure to apply.
3. Move your fingers slowly around the breast in a circular or wedge pattern until you have thoroughly examined all of the breast. (See figures **A** and **B**) Creep the fingers slowly along, being careful not to allow any unexamined breast to slip through the fingers. You will feel a firm ridge at the lower curve of each breast. This is normal.

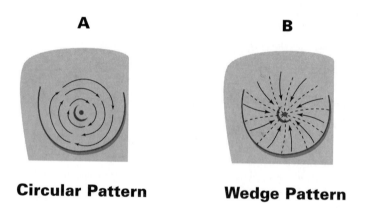

A   **B**

Circular Pattern   **Wedge Pattern**

4. Compress the nipple of each breast between thumb and index finger to observe for any discharge.

CONTINUE THE EXAMINATION

- Examine your breasts again while bathing. The slippery soap makes the fingers glide over the breasts making it easy to feel any changes.
- Examine the breasts while standing in front of the mirror, so you can visually follow the examination.

WHAT TO REPORT

- **Any changes or abnormal findings should be reported to your physician immediately.**

THE BESt TIME FOR BSE

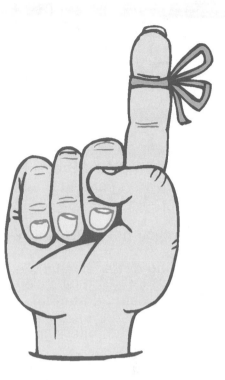

Breast Self Exam (BSE) should be performed monthly. It should be done at the same time each month. This is important, because in addition to examining for lumps, you want to compare how the breast feel from one month to the next to be aware of any changes. The difficult part of BSE is not the exam itself. **The difficult part of BSE is remembering to perform the exam.** It is easy to let the weeks pass by, and suddenly before you know it months have lapsed since the last exam.

The following tips are good ideas that will help you remember to perform BSE. But remembering to perform BSE is only half the challenge. The other half is actually performing the exam. IT COULD SAVE YOUR LIFE!

1. Pick a particular monthly utility bill that comes at the same time every month. When the bill arrives in the mail, that is the reminder to perform monthly breast self exam . . . on that day.

2. Choose the day of the month on which your birthday falls. For example: If your birthday falls on the tenth of May, the tenth of every month is the day to perform BSE. And the tenth of May of every year will be the day to see your physician for your annual check-up. What an easy way to remember your important breast exam and your annual check-up.

3. Many people have schedule or appointment books. If you have your days, weeks, or months scheduled in a book, write "BSE" on the first of every month for the entire year or the remaining calendar year. Do not strike through "BSE" until you have actually completed the exam.

4. If you have a sister(s), use the team approach. Whoever remembers and performs BSE first in the month is responsible for calling the other. At the end of the year, whoever has made the most "BSE" calls gets treated to an evening out by the other(s).

SCAVENGER HUNT BREAST EXAM

DIRECTIONS:

1. Locate on the diagram below the areas to be self-examined each month as you perform a Self-Breast Exam. Make an "X" on the picture below on the following parts of the female body: Clavicle (Collar Bone)   Axilla (Underarm)
Sternum (Breastbone)   Nipple

2. Outline the entire area to be examined with a solid line.

3. Using dotted lines draw the circular exam pattern on the left breast.

4. Next, using dotted lines draw the wedge pattern on the right breast.

5. Answer the following:

Name the positions for breast examination?

_____

How often should you examine your breasts?

_____

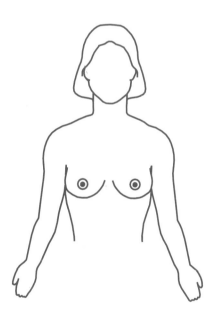

When, during the month, is the best time to examine your breasts?

_____

What are some of the ways you can remember to perform monthly BSE?

1. _____

2. _____

3. _____

What findings should you report to the doctor?

_____

_____

270

SCAVENGER HUNT BREAST EXAM

ANSWER KEY:

1. Locate on the diagram below the areas to be self-examined each month as you perform a Self-Breast Exam. Make an "X" on the picture on the following parts of the female body: Clavicle (Collar Bone)   Axilla (Underarm)
Sternum (Breastbone)   Nipple

2. Outline the entire area to be examined with a solid line.

3. Using dotted lines draw the circular exam pattern on the left breast.

4. Next, using dotted lines draw the wedge pattern on the right breast.

5. Answer the following: Name the positions for breast examination.

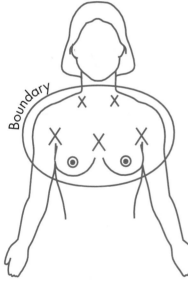

Arms hanging loosely at the sides; arms stretched out overhead; hands pressed together in front of chest; sitting; standing; leaning forward; lying on back

How often should you examine your breasts?

At least monthly

When, during the month, is the best time to examine your breasts?

7 to 10 days after your period; if you have no period, examine your breasts on the same day each month.

What are some of the ways you can remember to perform monthly BSE?

1. Select a utility bill that is received **monthly** and each month when the bill is received perform BSE.

2. Designate your birthday as **monthly** BSE day.

3. Choose a date 1–30—mark this date on **each month** of your calendar for the remaining months of the year. At the end of the year continue the same routine for the next year and so on.

What findings should you report to the doctor?

Report changes and abnormal findings to your doctor immediately.

271

THIS IS A STICK UP! AND PIGGIE AEROBICS

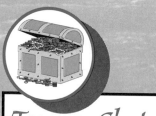

Treasure Chest

"This Is A Stick Up!" and "Piggie Aerobics"

Toy sheriff badge

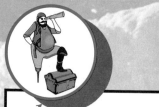

Educator Insights

Encourage the caregiver to remind the patient to keep feet propped up whenever possible.

PREPARATION

1. Copy and review "This Is A Stick Up!"
2. Copy and review "Piggie Aerobics."*

*Both "Treasures" may be used during a single visit or you may prefer to use them on separate visits.

IMPLEMENTATION

1. Review "This Is A Stick Up" with the patient.
2. Review "Piggie Aerobics" with the patient.
3. Wear a toy sheriff's badge during the visit. If you have an extra badge, award it to the caregiver, along with the authority to remind the patient of "This Is A Stick Up!"
4. Leave "This Is A Stick Up!" and "Piggie Aerobics" with the patient.

By: Gaye Ragland, RN, BSN

This is a Stick Up!

"Stick Up Your Feet"

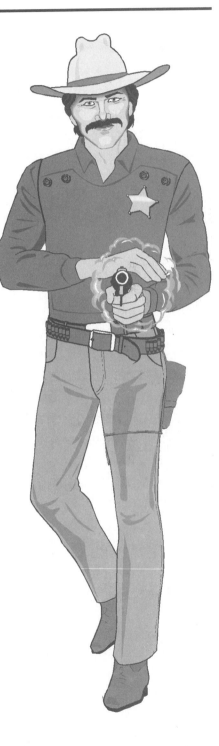

Because you have a history of swelling in your feet and legs, it is recommended that you keep your feet propped up during the day as you sit about. Circulation in the lower legs tends to often slow down with age and with certain other diseases. This can result in a build-up of fluid. Sitting or standing for long periods of time tends to worsen this problem of leg swelling.

When you are sitting during the day, it is recommended that you prop your feet on a footstool. Do not wear tight garters or socks. Avoid knee-hi stockings with snug bands. A helpful way to increase the circulation in your feet and lower legs is to perform foot and toe exercises throughout the day. They can be done any time during the day and may be done when you get up in the morning and when you go to bed at night. If you watch television throughout the day, it is a good practice to do the exercises during commercials. The exercises are easy to do. Simply bend your toes by curling and relaxing the toes. You may perform the exercises on both feet at the same time. Repeat the curling and relaxing of your toes at least five times on each foot. Then turn the foot and ankle clockwise five to ten times. Now reverse it, moving the foot and ankle in a counterclockwise direction for five to ten times. Repeat the foot and ankle exercises for the other foot. Rest between the foot exercises if you become tired.

273

"Piggie Aerobics"

As you sit around during the day, perform the following foot and toe exercises to keep the blood flowing and lessen the amount of fluid build-up in your feet and lower legs.

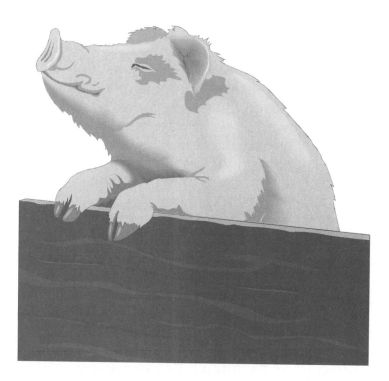

For your "little piggies" (toes):

Bend your toes by curling and relaxing the toes. You may exercise all of your toes at the same time. If you watch television during the day, a good way to remember to exercise is to repeat the exercise during the commercial breaks. Do "piggie aerobics" when you get up in the morning and when you go to bed at night.

For your "piggie holders" (feet):

Turn the left foot and ankle clockwise five to ten times. Now, turn the right foot and ankle clockwise five to ten times.

Now, repeat the exercises on each foot five to ten times, but this time turn the feet in a counterclockwise direction.

FOOTSTOOL CONSTRUCTION

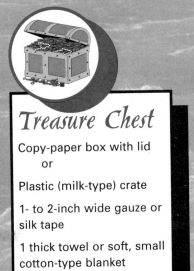

BUILDING A FOOTSTOOL

PREPARATION

1. Obtain standard size, sturdy copy-paper box with the original lid.
2. Obtain 1- to 2-inch silk or gauze tape.
3. Obtain a thick, soft towel or small, soft blanket from the patient to cover the footstool.

IMPLEMENTATION

1. Bring box, lid, and tape to the patient's home.
2. Obtain a thick, soft towel or small, soft blanket from the patient to cover the box.
3. If a blanket is offered, make the patient aware that the blanket will wrap the entire box. Get the patient's approval for the part of the blanket that covers the bottom of the box to be on the floor.
4. Tape the covering to the box. Secure by taping around the box and on both ends.

By: Gaye Ragland, RN, BSN

Treasure Chest

Copy-paper box with lid

or

Plastic (milk-type) crate

1- to 2-inch wide gauze or silk tape

1 thick towel or soft, small cotton-type blanket

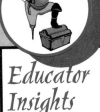

Educator Insights

You may offer the following tip to selected families: less expensive furniture stores carry a vinyl-covered stool for about $20.

Footstool Construction

Obtain a strong, standard size copy-paper box with the original, snugly-fitting lid. Tape the lid securely on the box. Pad the top of the box with at least one thick towel and tape the towel to the box with silk- or gauze-type tape. To add strength to the box, the patient may provide you with a small, cotton type blanket which may be wrapped around the entire box in the place of using the towel.

If available, a small plastic crate works well once it is padded for comfort. If a crate is not available, you may ask your local grocer to donate a small plastic milk crate (without revealing the patient's name, of course).

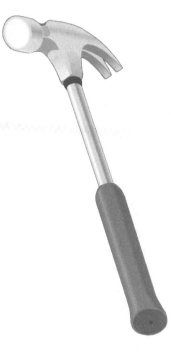

276

SIGNS OF THE TIMES

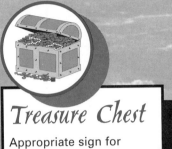

Treasure Chest

Appropriate sign for posting

Tape

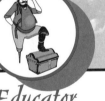

Educator Insights

Ask the patient or the patient's caregiver to post the sign in the desired location. They will know best which freshly painted walls or wallpaper to avoid.

PREPARATION

1. Copy the appropriate sign needed for posting.

IMPLEMENTATION

1. Obtain permission to post the appropriate sign.
2. Determine the best location for the sign to be posted.
3. Assist the patient or the patient's caregiver to post the sign.

By: Gaye Ragland, RN, BSN

DON'T FORGET YOUR DOCTOR'S APPOINTMENT

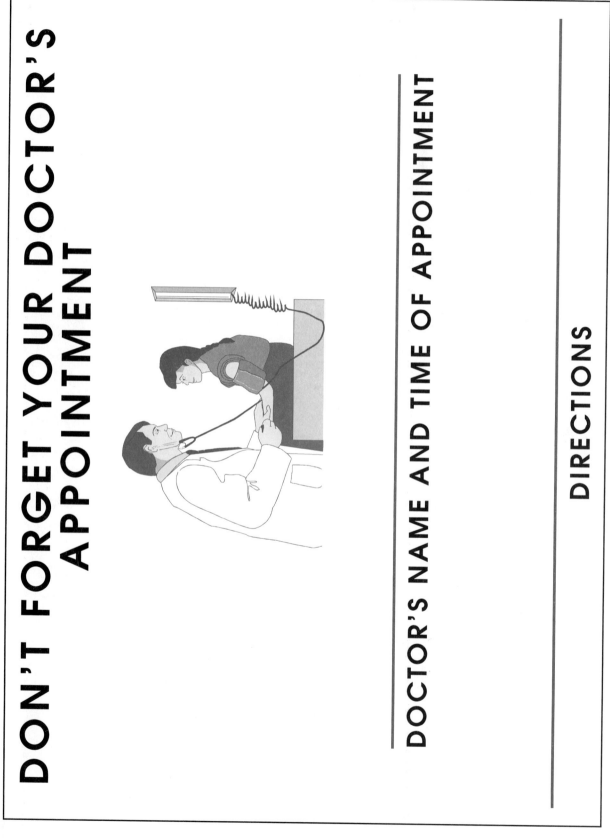

DOCTOR'S NAME AND TIME OF APPOINTMENT

DIRECTIONS

278

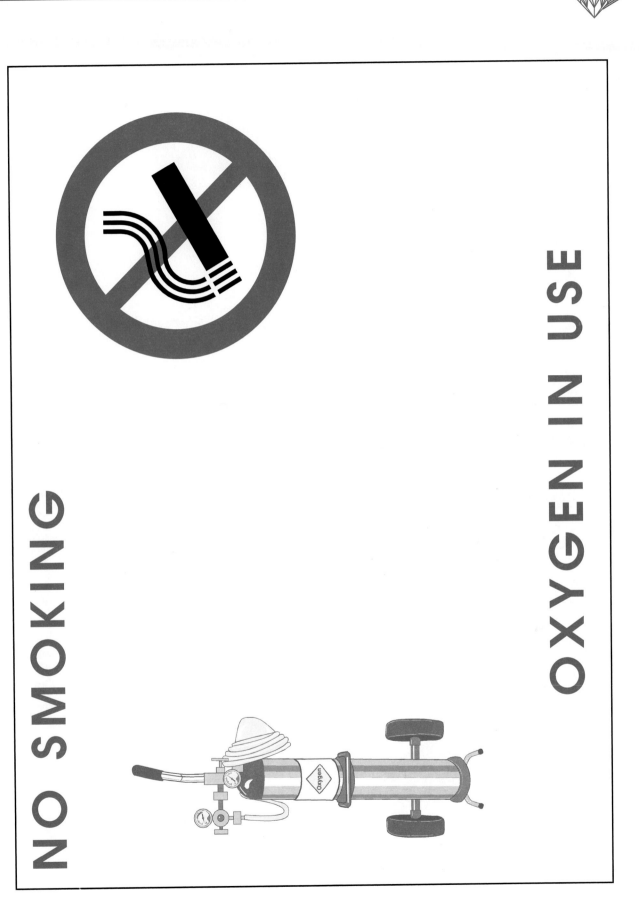

NO SMOKING

OXYGEN IN USE

279

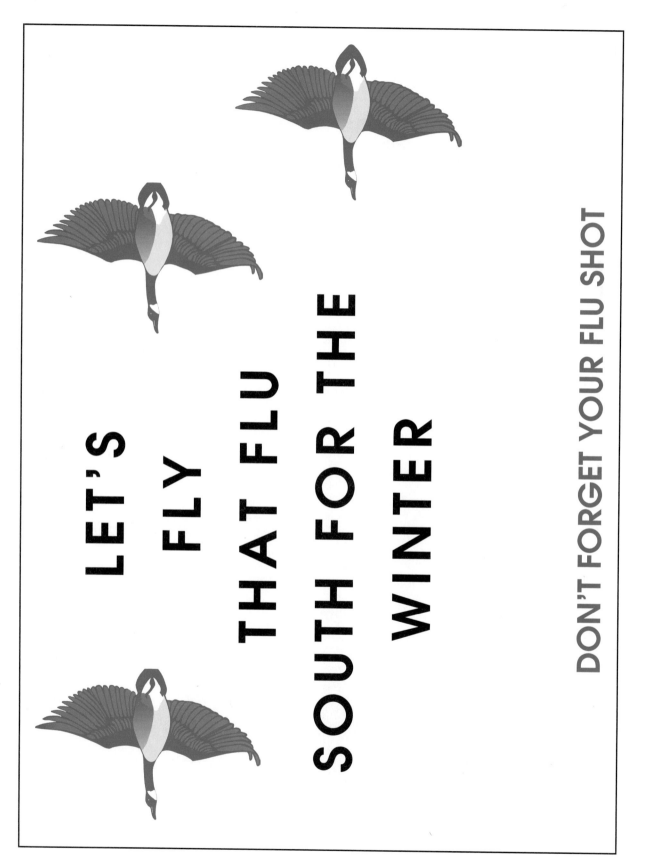

LET'S
FLY
THAT FLU
SOUTH FOR THE
WINTER

DON'T FORGET YOUR FLU SHOT

280

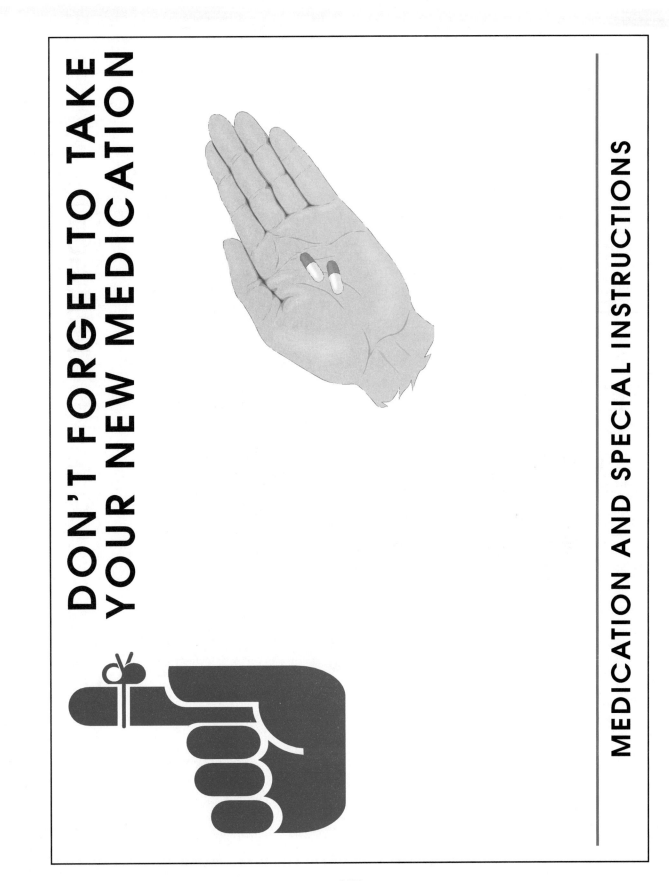

DON'T FORGET TO TAKE YOUR NEW MEDICATION

MEDICATION AND SPECIAL INSTRUCTIONS

WHEN RESTING ON YOUR SEAT

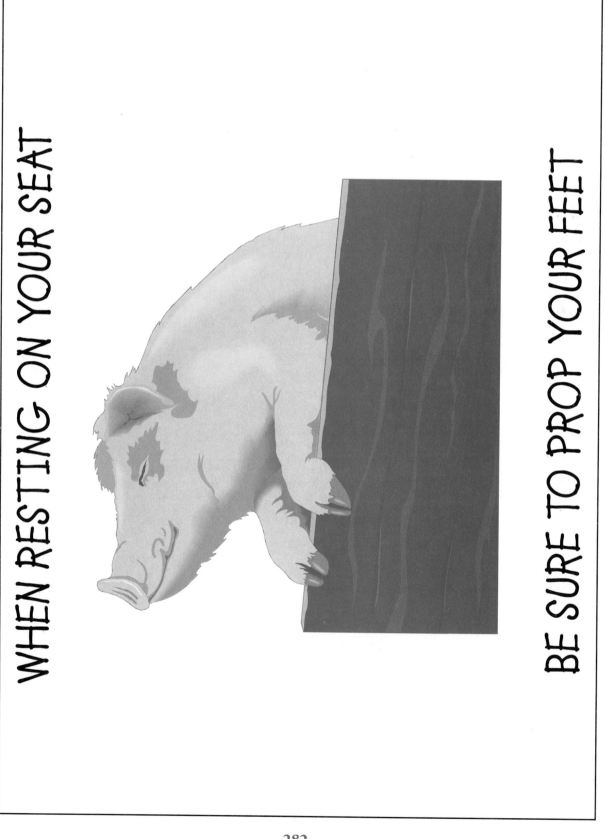

BE SURE TO PROP YOUR FEET

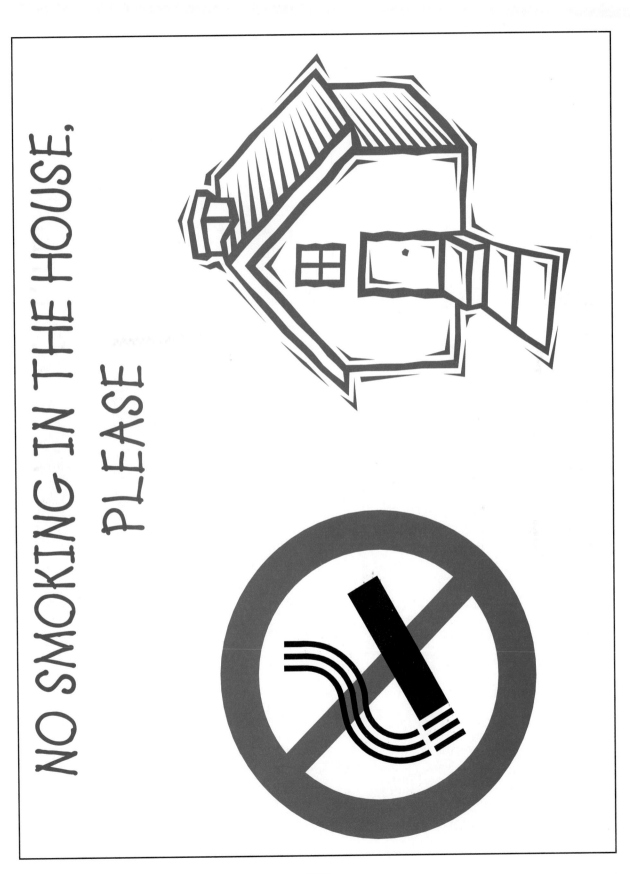

NO SMOKING IN THE HOUSE, PLEASE

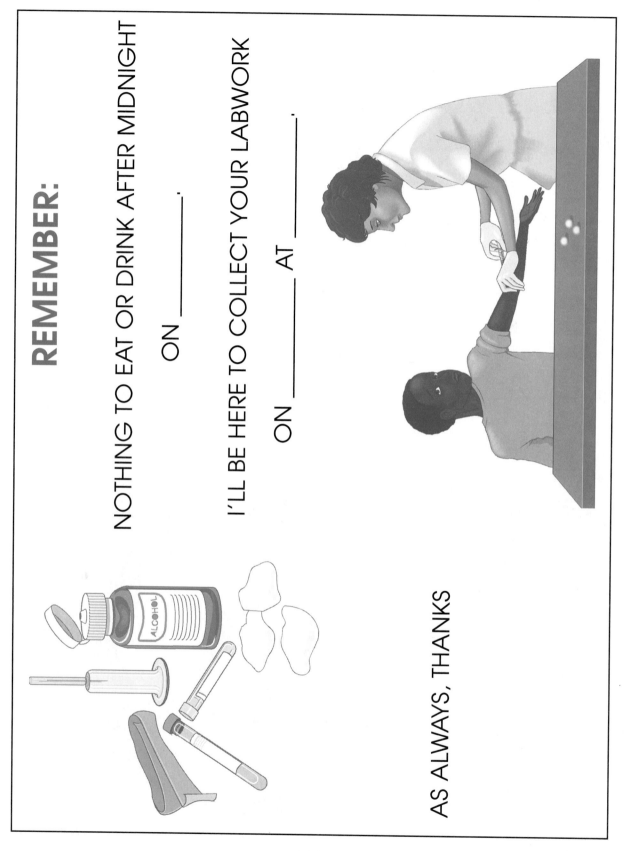

REMEMBER:

NOTHING TO EAT OR DRINK AFTER MIDNIGHT

ON _____.

I'LL BE HERE TO COLLECT YOUR LABWORK

ON _____ AT _____.

AS ALWAYS, THANKS

284

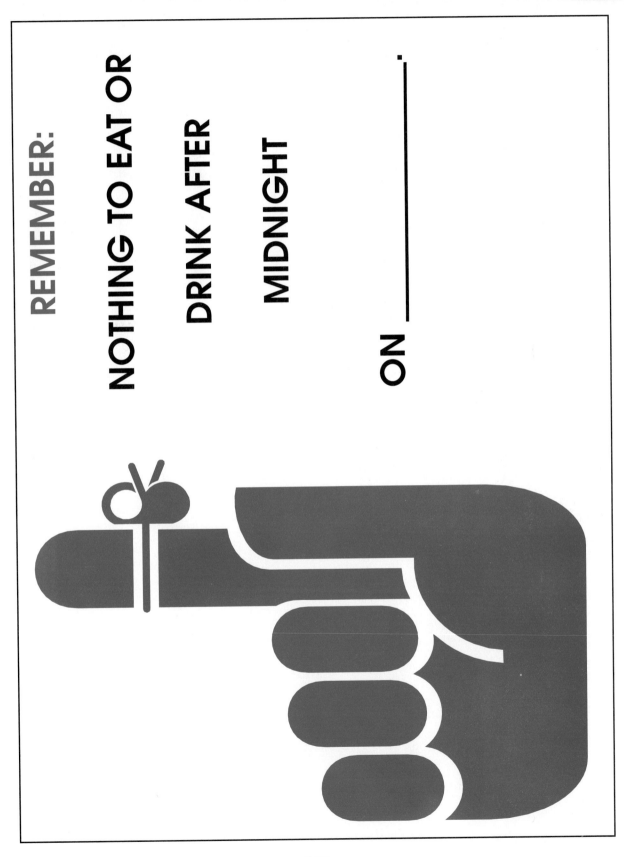

REMEMBER:

NOTHING TO EAT OR
DRINK AFTER
MIDNIGHT

ON _____.

285

HELP . . . HELP . . . HELP . . . HELP . . . HELP

Do you have an idea for an Instant Patient Teaching Treasure? If you would like to contribute a treasure for Volume II of *Instant Patient Teaching Treasures,* please complete the template on the following page. You may make as many copies of the instruction template as you like and send the completed form(s) to:

Gaye Ragland
c/o Mosby
ATTN: Senior Manager
Division of Continuing Education and Training
11830 Westline Industrial Drive
St. Louis, MO 63146

name of treasure

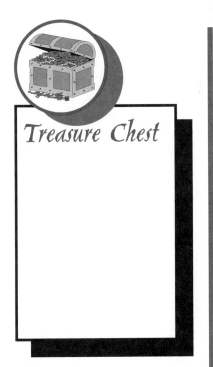

Treasure Chest

Educator Insights

PREPARATION

IMPLEMENTATION

By:

287

REFERENCES

American Heart Association Pamphlets as follows:
  About High Blood Pressure Control Risk Lifestyle Weight 50-1079, 1993, 1995
  Cholesterol And Your Heart 50-1059 (CP), 1989, 1992, 1993, 1995
  Controlling Your Risk Factors for Heart Attack 50-1062, 1993
  The Heart and Blood Vessels 50-0001 (CP)
  Heart and Stroke Facts 55-0519, 1992, 1993, 1994
  Heart and Stroke Facts 55-0521, 1995
  Heart Quiz 51-012 A, 1994.
  High Blood Pressure In African-Americans 50-1078, 1995
  Tips for Eating Out 50-1073, 1995
  Salt, Sodium and Blood Pressure 50-065B, 1979
  Smoking and Heart Disease 51-1057 (CP), 1986, 1992, 1995

Abrigani CA, Messenger B: *Alzheimer's disease: Activities that work,* La Grange, Texas, 1991, M & H.

Barnwell M, Kimball R, Raskopf V, Tapler D: *Diabetes,* El Paso, Texas, 1995, Skidmore-Roth.

Dantone J: *Bridging the Gap Procedure and Instructional Manual for Dietary and Nursing Interventions,* Grenada, Mississippi, 1993.

Beare P, Myers JL: *Adult Health Nursing,* ed 2, St. Louis, 1994, Mosby.

Castillo H: *The Nurse Assistant In Long Term Care: A Rehabilitative Approach,* St. Louis, 1992, Mosby.

Deck ML: *Instant Teaching Tools for Health Care Educators,* St Louis, 1995, Mosby.

Ebersole P, Hess P: *Toward Healthy Aging,* ed 4, St Louis, 1994, Mosby.

Elipoulos C: *Gerontological Nursing,* ed 2, Philadelphia, 1987, J. B. Lippincott.

Lambert S, Schneidman R, Wander BR: *Being A Nursing Assistant,* ed 6, Englewood Cliffs, NJ, 1991, Brady.

Long B, Phipps W, Cassmeyer V: *Medical-Surgical Nursing,* ed 3, St Louis, 1993, Mosby.

Mahan K, Arlin M: *Krause's Food, Nutrition and Diet Therapy,* ed 8, Philadelphia, 1992, W. B. Saunders Co.

Mayer KS: Managing the combative demented resident, *Nursing Homes* 43: 41–42, 1994.

Meyers D: *Client Teaching Guides for Home-Health Care,* Maryland, 1989, Aspen.

Miller C: *Nursing Care of Older Adults,* ed 2, Philadelphia, 1995, J. B. Lippincott.

Mixon MJ: Information Sheet #1462 "Safe Food Handling" and Information Sheet #1204 "Safe Food In A Hurry," Cooperative Extension Service/Mississippi State University/U. S. Department of Agriculture.

Potter P, Perry A: *Fundamentals of Nursing,* ed 3, St. Louis, 1993: Mosby.

Reader's Digest: Eat Better, Live Better A Common Sense Guide To Nutrition and Good Health, Pleasantville, NY, 1982, Reader's Digest Association, Inc.

Rice R: *Home Health Nursing Practice,* Philadelphia, 1992, Mosby.

Rice R: *Manual of Home Health Nursing Procedures,* St. Louis, 1995, Mosby.

Sandel S, Possidente E: The social re-enactment model for treating Alzheimer's disease, *Long-Term Care Administration* 21: 17–24, 1993–1994, Winter.

Schrefer S, editor: *Patient Teaching Guides* (1995). St. Louis, Mosby.

Smith S, Duall D: *Clinical Nursing Skills,* Norwalk, Connecticut, 1996, Appleton and Lange.

Sorrentino S: *Mosby's Textbook for Nursing Assistants,* ed 3, St. Louis, 1993, Mosby.

Stanley M, Beare P: *Gerontological Nursing,* Philadelphia, 1995, F. A. Davis.

Swearinggen P: *Manual of Medical Surgical Nursing Care Nursing Interventions and Collaborative Management,* ed 3, St Louis, 1994, Mosby.

Wardlaw G, Insel P, Seyler MF: *Contemporary Nutrition: Issues and Insights,* ed 2, St. Louis, 1994, Mosby.

U. S. Product Safety Commission: *Safety for Older Consumers: Home Safety Checklist,* Washington, D.C. 20207.

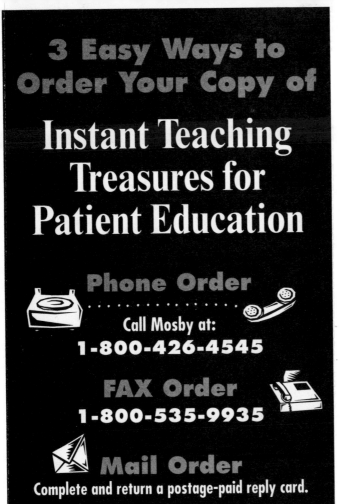
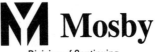
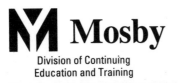

3 Easy Ways to Order Your Copy of

Instant Teaching Treasures for Patient Education

Phone Order

Call Mosby at:
1-800-426-4545

FAX Order
1-800-535-9935

Mail Order

Complete and return a postage-paid reply card.